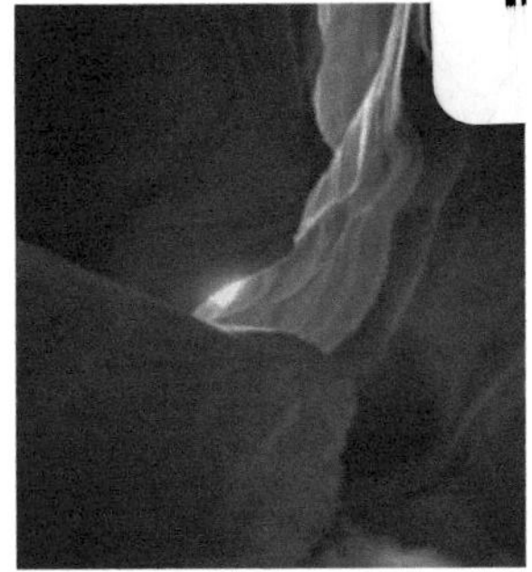

*You want*

*Your weight loss*

*Journey*

*To be*

*Sustainable,*

*Effortless*

*and*

*Personalized.*

*Period!*

*When you can see cause and effect*

*immediately,*

*making healthy*

*choices become intuitive*

*rather than*

*forced*

# The Glucose Reset:

*Effortless Weight Loss with CGM Technology*

**By Sudipta Mitra**

-

## Copyright & Legal Information

**The Glucose Reset: Effortless Weight Loss with CGM Technology**



**ISBN:** 979-8-9949526-0-3

**Edition:** 2026

**Intellectual Property Notice**

**Trademark Notice**



-

# Medical Disclaimer

## Important Health Information

This book is designed to provide information about using Continuous Glucose Monitors (CGMs) for weight loss and metabolic health. It is sold with the understanding that the author and publisher are not engaged in rendering medical, health, or any other kind of personal professional services in this book.

**This book is NOT medical advice.**

The content in this book is for educational and informational purposes only and should not be considered a substitute for professional medical advice, diagnosis, or treatment. Always seek the advice of your physician or other qualified health provider with any questions you may have regarding a medical condition or health objectives.

## Specific Warnings and Disclaimers

**Consult Your Healthcare Provider:** Before starting any new diet, exercise program, supplement regimen, or using a Continuous Glucose Monitor, you must consult with your physician or qualified healthcare provider, especially if you: -

- Have diabetes or prediabetes
- Are taking any medications

- Have any chronic health conditions
- Are pregnant or nursing
- Have a history of eating disorders

  CGM-based food tracking can reinforce obsessive thinking about food and eating. If you have a history of disordered eating, restrictive eating, or food anxiety, please consult a healthcare provider or eating disorder specialist before using a CGM for weight management.
- Are under 18 years of age

**Individual Results May Vary:** The strategies, suggestions, and information contained in this book are based on the author's research and published scientific literature. Success stories and examples presented in Chapter 10 are composite illustrations representing common patterns and outcomes, not specific real individuals. Results will vary based on individual circumstances, metabolism, genetics, adherence to protocols, and many other factors. There is no guarantee that you will experience the same results.

**Not a Diabetes Management Guide:** This book is intended for individuals without diabetes who are using CGM technology for metabolic optimization and weight loss. If you have diabetes or prediabetes, you must work with your healthcare team and follow their medical guidance. The target glucose ranges and protocols in this book may not be appropriate for individuals with diabetes.

**Technology Limitations:** CGM technology is continuously evolving. Information about specific devices, apps, and services may become outdated. Always refer to manufacturer instructions and current medical guidelines.

**Emergency Situations:** If you experience symptoms of hypoglycemia (very low blood sugar) such as shakiness, confusion, rapid heartbeat, or loss of consciousness, seek immediate medical attention. If you have any medical emergency, call emergency services immediately.

**Supplement Caution:** Any supplements mentioned in this book are for informational purposes only. Some supplements can interact with medications or may not be appropriate for certain individuals. Always consult your healthcare provider before starting any supplement.

**Liability Limitation:** The author and publisher shall have neither liability nor responsibility to any person or entity with respect to any loss, damage, or injury caused or alleged to be caused directly or indirectly by the information contained in this book.

**Assumption of Risk**

By reading and implementing any information from this book, you acknowledge that you are doing so at your own risk. You acknowledge that the author is not a licensed medical professional, and the information provided does not replace professional medical advice, diagnosis, or treatment.

**If you do not wish to be bound by this disclaimer and these terms, you may return this book for a full refund in accordance with the retailer's return policy.**

–

## Publisher's Note

Every effort has been made to ensure that the information contained in this book is complete and accurate at the time of publication. However, medical knowledge and technology are constantly evolving. The publisher and author cannot guarantee that the information will remain current or that it is suitable for every individual situation. Readers are encouraged to verify information with current medical literature and consult healthcare professionals for personalized advice.

-

## Dedication

To My Father and Mother

-

## Acknowledgments

Mrs. Sangita Mitra – who supported in my journey

Dr. Deepshikha Chowdhury – who suggested the Quick Start section

Mr. Sudhir Chelliru – who reviewed the first draft and started his own journey

Mr. Somdutta Sanyal – Who provided valuable suggestions with his thoroughness

Mr. Pratim Chowdhury – For His encouragement when starting the book

-

CONTENTS

Foreword....................XIII
Introduction: A New Lens on Weight Loss.......... XX

PART 1: QUICK START GUIDE....................1

Start Your Transformation TODAY!....................1
Hey there, Future You!....................1
Is This Guide for You?....................1
What You Need to Get Started.................... 2
SUCCESS STORIES.................... 5
Four dimensions, six daily practices — one goal. The 6 Golden Rules (THIS IS ALL YOU NEED).............. 10
A Note on Walking Alternatives....................13
YOUR 30-DAY TRANSFORMATION PLAN.............. 29
VISUAL TRANSFORMATION TIMELINE.............. 35
THE SUGGESTED FOOD GUIDE.................... 36
SUGGESTED DAILY SCHEDULE TEMPLATE.......... 38
THE 20-MINUTE WORKOUT....................41
TROUBLESHOOTING GUIDE.................... 44
SUGGESTED YOUR QUICK REFERENCE CHECKLIST .................... 49
KEY TAKEAWAYS....................51
YOUR NEXT STEPS.................... 52
FINAL PEP TALK.................... 53
ONE LAST THING.................... 54

PART 2: THE SCIENCE.................... 56

Deep Dive into The Science and Strategy.............. 56
Chapter 1: Understanding Continuous Glucose Monitors....................57

CHAPTER 2: THE GLUCOSE-WEIGHT CONNECTION..........58
CHAPTER 3: YOUR FIRST TWO WEEKS WITH A CGM........ 61
CHAPTER 4: READING YOUR CGM DATA ........................64
CHAPTER 5: THE 10 PRINCIPLES OF CGM-BASED WEIGHT LOSS ..........................................................................89
CHAPTER 6: COMMON CGM INSIGHTS FOR WEIGHT LOSS ........................................................................... 117
CHAPTER 7: BUILDING YOUR CGM-BASED WEIGHT LOSS PLAN ..................................................................... 124
CHAPTER 8: TROUBLESHOOTING COMMON CHALLENGES ........................................................................... 127
CHAPTER 9: BEYOND WEIGHT LOSS - LONG-TERM METABOLIC HEALTH .................................................. 130
CHAPTER 10: MAINTAINING YOUR SUCCESS................. 134
CHAPTER 11: SUCCESS STORIES AND PRACTICAL EXAMPLES ........................................................................... 137
CONCLUSION: YOUR METABOLIC JOURNEY ....................141
APPENDIX A: CGM QUICK REFERENCE GUIDE............. 144
APPENDIX B: WALKING ALTERNATIVES ....................... 145
APPENDIX C: RECOMMENDED RESOURCES.................... 152
APPENDIX D: ACRONYMS ............................................ 163
ABOUT THE AUTHOR......................................................171
ABOUT THIS BOOK AND ITS EVIDENCE......................... 172
WORKING ALONGSIDE YOUR HEALTHCARE TEAM ......... 172
ON GLP-1 MEDICATIONS AND THIS BOOK ................... 173
HOW CLAIMS ARE MADE IN THIS BOOK....................... 174
SLEEP AND INSULIN RESISTANCE................................. 175
POST-MEAL EXERCISE AND GLUCOSE SPIKES............... 176
FOOD SEQUENCING AND GLUCOSE RESPONSE .............. 176
DIABETES PREVENTION ...............................................177

# Foreword

## *You want your weight loss to be sustainable & effortless. Period!*

Tailor made diets & exercise plan help you lose weight, but has it been sustainable? Or how many of you have lost weight only to regain very quickly – I sure was one. Having been through such ups and downs my A1C one day hit 7.1.

*Author's note: An A1C of 7.1% meets the clinical threshold for a Type 2 diabetes diagnosis (≥6.5%). The author undertook this journey under medical supervision. This book is designed for individuals without diabetes or prediabetes; if you have a diagnosis or elevated A1C, please work with your healthcare provider before using CGM technology independently.*

## *I knew I had to do something about it*

I put the CGM on me and voila! I could see what spiked my glucose and what brought it back in real time - I was in control. Small changes in the meals I've been taking for years and bit of moving around. One metric changed everything.

The difference – I could SEE what was happening, so adjusted based on my personal data. And the result showed in 3 months I lost 20 pounds and was able to keep it at that. From being obese, though still now overweight, my A1C number is now 6.2 – not done yet but I know I can change at will. The best thing was that I just put CGM for 2 weeks, but my behavior changed forever, I was making better choices. At the end of 2 weeks I knew, what was good for my weight and what was not. I changed forever.

Two weeks was enough to rewire my instincts — but it was not the end of the journey. In the Quick Start Guide and the science chapters that follow, you will see how wearing your CGM across multiple phases (and returning to it periodically as your habits evolve) accelerates and deepens the learning. Think of two weeks as your proof of concept; think of the longer program as your transformation. The data you collect beyond those first two weeks is what turns fleeting insight into permanent, personalized habit.

**Individual results vary. The author's experience reflects outcomes achieved with medical supervision and may not be typical. Weight loss results depend on many factors including starting health status, adherence, metabolism, and individual circumstances. **

**Note**: "The CGM was my superpower. I could SEE what foods were sabotaging me and how exercise affected the readings. Once I saw it, I couldn't unsee it. *Game changer!*"

*Now that's personalized sustainable weight loss!*

*You are in control of your body, your data, your choice*

# *Don't look back. Gain control effortlessly.*

The book contains the learnings from my journey that will help you define your journey for personalized sustainable weight loss. Try it, would love to hear your own.

## THE FIRST WEEK

Putting on the CGM (please consult your primary care physician), I used a Lingo device, but I didn't know what to expect. But the app has a 'getting started' guide. You can use the device of your choice.

It started transmitting the reading after one hour. The first few days I was obsessed with the reading, slightest bumps would send me moving or eating less. Now that's not needed. The first week is to see how you are with your current way of life, around your diet & exercise (think movement) and start making minor adjustments on food choices, taking a walk after meals. I went to a party on the $2^{nd}$ day, and my glucose hit ~194 mg/dL. Not to worry, you learn from your mistakes don't you! That sets you up for course correction. I walked briskly for about 30 minutes after lunch and dinner (about 60 minutes total per day) and happily watched my glucose go back to the healthy range. The morning walk after breakfast was harder for me to fit in consistently given work meetings and family obligations, so I focused on the two meals I could control. This realistic approach worked perfectly. Both brought my glucose back into range; the 30-minute post-meal structure was easier to maintain long-term. Having reduced portions and balanced plates naturally helped.

## THE SECOND WEEK

This is when I experimented with my meals to include healthy fat, protein, and less carbs. What seemed to matter most is that I ate a balanced meal with a controlled portion and took regular walks after my two major meals—lunch and dinner—for about 30 minutes each, totaling about 60 minutes of walking per day. Each walk session would end when I took the last lap after having started to sweat. Purposeful, not strolling—you can talk but should feel slightly breathless, heart rate elevated but comfortable, about 3-4 mph. The app kept showing the glucose downward slide during the walk. This ONE METRIC DROVE my choice and unknowingly, without trying, I started losing weight.

**Note:** While I walked after two meals (lunch and dinner), the book presents the ideal protocol of walking after all three meals. Choose what's realistic for YOUR schedule—even one post-meal walk makes a significant difference.

## THIRD WEEK ONWARDS

The CGM device was taken off, but I couldn't UNSEE how my choices in the 4 dimensions of weight loss diet, activity, sleep & stress management that impacted my glucose.

*My weight loss journey*

*became sustainable*

*based on my personal data,*

*it could be your story too*

## Introduction: A New Lens on Weight Loss

For decades, we've approached weight loss the same way: count calories, exercise more, eat less. Yet obesity rates continue to climb, and most dieters regain their lost weight within a few years. What if we've been looking at the problem through the wrong lens?

Continuous Glucose Monitors (CGMs) offer a revolutionary new perspective on weight loss—one that focuses not on how much you eat, but on how your body responds to what you eat. Originally designed for people with diabetes, these small wearable sensors are now revealing profound insights about metabolism, hunger, energy, and fat storage in everyone.

*Cost and accessibility note: Consumer CGM sensors typically cost $75–$150+ per sensor (each lasts 10–14 days). Health insurance does not generally cover CGM use for non-diabetic wellness purposes. The author used* **Lingo by Abbott** (hellolingo.com). CGM availability and whether a prescription is required varies by country and region — search "CGM for wellness" in your local search engine to find options near you.

## The Four Dimensions of Effortless Weight Loss

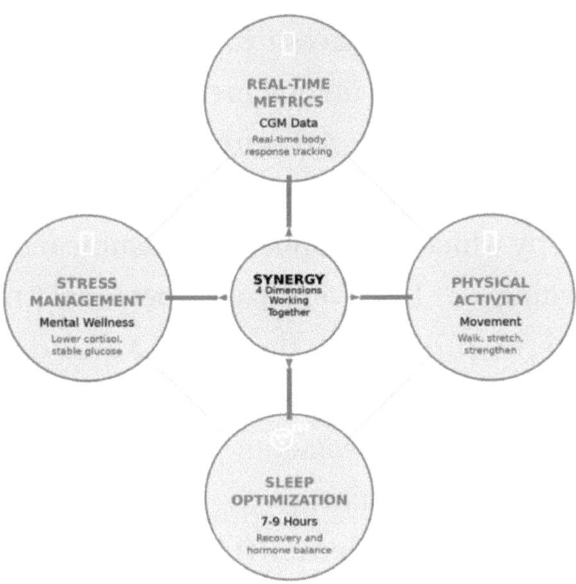


## Introduction: A New Lens on Weight Loss

True effortless weight loss isn't about willpower or deprivation—it's about aligning four critical dimensions that work synergistically to transform your metabolism and your body. This book is built on these foundational pillars:

*1. Real-Time Metrics-Driven Approach*

**Why It Matters**: For the first time in human history, you can see exactly how your body responds to food, stress, sleep, and activity in real-time. No more guessing. No more generic diet advice. Just your unique metabolic data.

**The CGM Advantage**: - See glucose responses within minutes of eating - Identify exactly which foods spike your insulin and block fat burning - Discover your personal metabolic patterns throughout the day - Make data-driven decisions instead of following one-size-fits-all rules - Track improvements objectively as your metabolism transforms

**Effortless Element**: When you can see cause and effect immediately, making healthy choices becomes intuitive rather than forced. You're not following rules—you're responding to your body's clear signals.

*2. Stress Management*

**Why It Matters**: Chronic stress elevates cortisol, which directly raises blood glucose, promotes insulin resistance, and triggers fat storage—especially dangerous belly fat. Your CGM may show you that stress raises your glucose even without eating — in some people, psychological stress produces a measurable glucose rise as the body mobilizes energy for the perceived threat. The magnitude varies considerably between individuals.

**The Comprehensive Approach**:

- Understanding the stress-glucose-cortisol connection
- Practical stress reduction techniques that lower glucose
- The journey from self-criticism to self-compassion
- Breaking free from the stress of perfectionism
- Building a peaceful relationship with food and your body

**Effortless Element**: When you manage stress, cravings decrease, energy stabilizes, and weight loss happens naturally without the constant mental battle. You're working with your nervous system, not against it.

*3. Sleep Optimization*

**Why It Matters**: Poor sleep is one of the fastest ways to derail weight loss. Even a single night of inadequate sleep can meaningfully increase insulin resistance, raise fasting glucose the next day, intensify cravings for high-carb foods, and slow your metabolism. A controlled study at the University of Chicago found approximately 30% reduced insulin sensitivity after sleep restriction — a striking finding, though based on a small sample under specific lab conditions. The direction of the effect is well established and consistently replicated. [Spiegel et al., 1999, The Lancet; Leproult & Van Cauter, 2010, JAMA]

**The Sleep-Glucose Connection**:

- Your CGM reveals how sleep quality affects next-day glucose control
- Sleep deprivation raises cortisol and glucose even without eating
- Deep sleep is when your body repairs and optimizes metabolism
- Consistent sleep schedules synchronize circadian rhythms with insulin sensitivity
- Quality sleep reduces hunger hormones and enhances fat burning

**Effortless Element**: When you're well-rested, you naturally make better food choices, have stable energy, and experience fewer cravings. Weight loss becomes easier because your hormones are balanced and your willpower isn't depleted.

*4. Physical Activity*

**Why It Matters**: Movement isn't just about burning calories—it's about improving insulin sensitivity, helping muscles absorb glucose without requiring insulin, and creating metabolic flexibility. Your CGM will show you the immediate glucose-lowering effects of even gentle movement.

**The Strategic Approach**:

- Post-meal walks/movement that dramatically reduce glucose spikes
- Strength training that improves glucose disposal for 24-48 hours
- Activity timing to maximize metabolic benefits
- Finding movement, you enjoy rather than forcing exercise you hate
- Building sustainable activity habits into your daily routine

**Effortless Element**: When you see your glucose curve flatten in real-time during a walk, movement becomes rewarding rather than punishing. You're not exercising to "burn off" food—you're optimizing your metabolism.

**The Synergistic Power of Integration**

Here's what makes this approach truly effortless: these four dimensions don't just add to each other—they multiply each other's effects.

**The Positive Spiral**: - Better sleep → lower stress → better glucose control → easier to exercise

- More movement → better sleep → lower cortisol → improved insulin sensitivity

- Stress management → better food choices → stable glucose → deeper sleep

- Real-time metrics → clear feedback → reduced anxiety → better decisions

When all four dimensions align, weight loss stops being a battle and becomes a natural outcome. You're not forcing your body to change through deprivation and willpower—you're creating the conditions where your body naturally returns to health.

**The Truth About Lifestyle Change: It's All About Behavior**

You've probably heard that weight loss is a "lifestyle change," not a diet. While this sounds inspiring, it often feels vague and overwhelming. What does it mean to change your lifestyle?

**The Reality**: At its core, sustainable weight loss is about changing a specific set of behaviors and repeating them consistently until they become automatic—until they simply become who you are.

**From Conscious Effort to Unconscious Identity**:

Every behavior you currently have—whether it's reaching for a snack when stressed, scrolling through your phone before bed, or skipping breakfast—started as a conscious choice. Repeated over time, these choices became habits. Repeated longer, they became your lifestyle. They're now so automatic you don't even think about them.

The good news? This same process works in reverse and in your favor.

**The Behavioral Transformation Journey**:

1. **Awareness** (Weeks 1-2): You consciously notice your current patterns through CGM data. "I always spike after my morning muffin." This is observation without judgment.
2. **Experimentation** (Weeks 3-6): You deliberately try new behaviors. "What if I eat eggs instead?" This requires conscious effort and feels awkward at first.
3. **Practice** (Weeks 7-12): The new behaviors become easier with repetition. "I automatically reach for eggs now." You still think about it, but it's becoming natural.

**Integration** (Months 4-6): The behaviors feel normal. "This is just what I eat for breakfast." You rarely think about the old way.

4. **Identity** (Months 6+): The behaviors have become part of who you are. "I'm someone who eats protein for breakfast." It's no longer something you do—it's someone you are.

**Why This Matters for "Effortless" Weight Loss**:

The word "effortless" doesn't mean you never put in effort—it means you put in effort strategically at the beginning, so that the behaviors eventually become automatic and truly require minimal ongoing effort.

Think about brushing your teeth. It probably feels effortless now. You don't agonize over whether to brush, you don't need willpower, you don't negotiate with yourself. You just do it. But as a child learning this behavior, it required reminders, effort, and consistency. Now it's simply part of your identity as someone who brushes their teeth.

**The same transformation happens with metabolic health behaviors**:

- Checking your CGM after meals becomes as automatic as checking your phone

- Taking a post-dinner walk becomes as routine as brushing your teeth
- Eating protein first becomes as natural as putting on your seatbelt
- Choosing foods that stabilize your glucose becomes as obvious as avoiding foods, you're allergic to

**The CGM Accelerates This Process**:

What makes CGM technology so powerful is that it dramatically speeds up the journey from conscious behavior to automatic habit. Here's how:

**Immediate Feedback**: Instead of waiting weeks or months to see results on a scale, you see the impact of your choices within days. This tight feedback loop strengthens new behaviors quickly.

**Personal Relevance**: You're not following someone else's rules—you're responding to your own body's signals. Behaviors that are personally meaningful stick better than generic advice.

**Intrinsic Motivation**: When you see your glucose stabilize and feel your energy improve, you want to continue the behavior. It's rewarding, not just a means to an end.

**Reduced Decision Fatigue**: Once you know which foods work for your metabolism, you stop debating. The decision is made. This preserves willpower for other areas of life.

**The Long Game: Behavior Becomes Life**: The goal isn't to track your glucose forever or to think about food constantly for the rest of your life. The goal is to build a set of behaviors so deeply ingrained that they become your default way of living.

You want to reach the point where:

- You instinctively choose foods that serve your body
- Movement is a natural part of your day, not a scheduled obligation
- Stress management practices happen automatically when you need them - good sleep hygiene is just "how you do bedtime"
- These behaviors feel like you, not like something you're doing

**This is when weight loss becomes permanent**. Not because you're following a diet, but because you've fundamentally changed the behaviors that created excess weight in the first place. The weight stays off because the person who created that weight no longer exists—you've become someone else, someone whose natural behaviors maintain a healthy weight.

**The Beautiful Paradox**:

Here's the beautiful paradox of this approach: you must be very intentional and conscious at the beginning—tracking, logging, experimenting, learning. It feels like a lot of work. But you're doing this work specifically so that eventually, you don't have to work at it anymore.

You're building a foundation of behaviors that will serve you for decades with minimal ongoing effort. You're investing in becoming the kind of person for whom healthy choices are the default, not the exception.

**Starting Your Behavioral Transformation**:

As you read this book, remember you're not just learning about glucose or trying a new diet. You're beginning a behavioral transformation that will compound over time. Every small action you take based on your CGM data is a brick in the foundation of your new identity.

Be patient with the process. Be compassionate with yourself as you learn. And trust that with consistency, what feels difficult and deliberate today will eventually feel effortless and automatic.

That's when you'll know you haven't just lost weight—you've truly changed your life.

This book is built on four interconnected dimensions — real-time metrics, strategic movement, sleep optimization, and stress management — expressed as six daily practices you will find in the Quick Start Guide. Master the practices and you are, by definition, mastering the dimensions.

## If You Do Nothing Else, Do These Six Things

If the comprehensive approach in this book feels overwhelming, or if you simply want to know the absolute essentials that deliver the most impact, here are the six non-negotiables. These are the behaviors that, if practiced consistently, will transform your metabolic health and lead to sustainable weight loss—even if you ignore everything else:

*1. Take a Brisk 30-Minute Walk After Every Major Meal*

**Why This Matters Most**: This single habit combines glucose control, stress reduction, and physical activity in one simple action. Research shows that post-meal walking consistently and significantly reduces glucose spikes and the associated insulin response compared to staying seated — making it one of the most effective and accessible tools for metabolic health. [Colberg et al., 2009, Diabetes Care; Reynolds et al., 2016, Diabetologia]

**The Complete Protocol - Three Tiers:**

TIER 1: IDEAL (90 minutes/day)

Walk 30 minutes after breakfast, lunch, AND dinner.

→ This is the gold standard for maximum glucose control and fastest weight loss.

TIER 2: EFFECTIVE (60 minutes/day) WHAT I ACTUALLY DID

Walk 30 minutes after lunch AND dinner (skip breakfast walk if needed).

→ This is what I personally did to lose 20 pounds. Post-lunch and post-dinner walks were my non-negotiables. The morning walk was often impossible due to work meetings, school drop-offs, and early commitments. Focusing on TWO consistent walks worked perfectly.

TIER 3: MINIMUM (30 minutes/day)

Walk 30 minutes after dinner only.

→ If you can only do ONE walk, make it after dinner. Evening glucose elevation has the most negative impact on overnight fat burning, morning fasting glucose, and sleep quality.

"Choose the tier that fits YOUR life. Tier 2 (lunch + dinner) is a realistic, sustainable approach that delivers excellent results—I'm living proof.

**Examples**:

**After Breakfast (30 minutes)**:

- Walk around your neighborhood before starting work
- Walk while taking a phone call
- Park farther from your office and walk the rest
- Use a treadmill desk or walking pad while checking emails
- Walk your kids to school instead of driving

**After Lunch (30 minutes)**:

- Take a walking meeting with colleagues
- Walk to a nearby park and back during your lunch break
- Walk to get your lunch instead of delivery
- Walk around your office building or parking lot
- Use stairs instead of elevators for your full break

**After Dinner (30 minutes)**:
- Walk with your spouse or partner—make it conversation time
- Walk your dog (or offer to walk a neighbor's dog)
- Listen to a podcast or audiobook while walking
- Walk to a nearby destination (coffee shop, friend's house)
- Evening walk with the family as a wind-down ritual

**Total Daily Walking**: 90 minutes across three meals. This may sound like a lot, but it's broken into manageable chunks and happens when you're naturally taking a break anyway (after eating).

**The Key**: "Brisk" means purposeful, not strolling. You should be able to talk but feel slightly breathless. This intensity activates muscles to absorb glucose.

**Start Small If Needed**: - **Week 1**: 10 minutes after each meal (30 min/day total) - **Week 2-3**: 15 minutes after each meal (45 min/day total) - **Week 4-5**: 20 minutes after each meal (60 min/day total) - **Week 6+**: 30 minutes after each meal (90 min/day total)

Even starting with 10 minutes after each meal provides measurable benefits on your CGM.

**If You Can Only Walk After One Meal**: Choose dinner. Evening glucose elevation has the most negative impact on overnight fat burning, morning fasting glucose, and sleep quality. But the goal is all three meals.

*2. Eat a Balanced Meal Every Time—And Control Your Portions*

**Why This Matters**: The composition of your meals directly determines your glucose response. A balanced plate stabilizes blood sugar, reduces insulin spikes, and naturally controls hunger. Your CGM will show you that what's ON your plate matters as much as how much is on it.

**The Glucose-Stable Plate Formula**:

Every meal should include all four components in the right proportions:

**1. Non-Starchy Vegetables (40-50% of your plate)** - Leafy greens: spinach, kale, lettuce, arugula - Cruciferous: broccoli, cauliflower, Brussels sprouts, cabbage - Other vegetables: bell peppers, zucchini, asparagus, green beans, tomatoes, cucumbers, mushrooms

**Why**: Fiber slows glucose absorption, provides volume without calories, and feeds beneficial gut bacteria that improve glucose metabolism.

**2. Protein (25-30% of your plate)**

- Animal sources: chicken, turkey, fish, eggs, lean beef, pork
- Plant sources: tofu, tempeh, legumes, lentils
- Dairy: Greek yogurt, cottage cheese

**Why**: Protein slows gastric emptying, reduces glucose spikes, increases satiety, and preserves muscle mass during weight loss. Muscle is metabolically active and improves glucose disposal.

**3. Healthy Fats (15-20% of your plate)**

- Avocado - Nuts and seeds (almonds, walnuts, chia, flax)
- Olive oil or avocado oil - Fatty fish (salmon, sardines, mackerel)
- Nut butters

**Why**: Fat further slows digestion and glucose absorption, increases satiety, and is essential for hormone production and nutrient absorption.

**4. Complex Carbohydrates (5-15% of your plate, optional)**

- Whole grains: quinoa, brown rice, steel-cut oats

- Starchy vegetables: sweet potato, butternut squash

- Legumes: lentils, chickpeas, black beans (double as protein)

- Fruits: berries (lower glycemic impact)

**Why**: When included in small amounts with fiber, protein, and fat, complex carbs provide energy without extreme glucose spikes. Many people find they need very little or can skip entirely for optimal glucose control.

**Practical Meal Examples**:

**Breakfast Option 1**:

- 3 eggs scrambled (protein)

- 1 cup sautéed spinach and mushrooms (vegetables)

- ½ avocado (healthy fat)

- Small handful of berries (optional carb)

**Breakfast Option 2**: - Greek yogurt, full-fat, plain (protein + fat)

- Handful of almonds (protein + fat)

- 1 cup mixed berries (carb)

- Chia seeds (fiber + fat)

**Lunch**: - Grilled chicken breast, 4-6 oz (protein)

- Large mixed green salad with cucumbers, tomatoes, peppers (vegetables)

- Olive oil and vinegar dressing (healthy fat)

- ½ cup quinoa (optional complex carb)

**Dinner**:

- Grilled salmon, 4-6 oz (protein + healthy fat)

- Roasted broccoli and cauliflower, 2 cups (vegetables)

- Side salad with olive oil (vegetables + fat)

- Small, sweet potato (optional complex carb)

**Portion Control: The Right Amount Matters**

Even balanced meals can spike glucose if portions are too large. Your CGM will teach you your personal portion limits.

**The Hand Method for Portion Control**: Easy Reference

- **Protein**: Palm-sized portion (about 4-6 oz or 20-30g protein)
- **Vegetables**: Two fists worth (unlimited non-starchy vegetables)
- **Healthy fats**: Thumb-sized portion (about 1-2 tablespoons)
- **Complex carbs**: Cupped hand or less (about ½ cup cooked)

**Start Larger, Then Adjust Based on CGM Data**:

1. **Week 1**: Eat your normal portions but in balanced ratios

2. **Monitor your CGM**: Note which meals spike you above 140 mg/dL
3. **Week 2-3**: Reduce portions of whatever caused spikes (usually carbs)
4. **Find your threshold**: The amount you can eat while staying under 130 mg/dL post-meal
5. **Lock it in**: Make these portions your new normal

**Common Portion Mistakes Your CGM Will Reveal**:

**Mistake 1: Too many carbs, even if "healthy"** - 1 cup of brown rice might spike you to 160 mg/dL - ½ cup keeps you at 120 mg/dL - Solution: Cut the carb portion in half

**Mistake 2: Not enough protein or fat** - Salad with grilled chicken but fat-free dressing: spike to 150 mg/dL - Same salad with olive oil dressing: spike to 115 mg/dL - Solution: Always include adequate fat

**Mistake 3: "Healthy" smoothies with too much fruit** - Smoothie with 2 bananas, berries, juice: spike to 170 mg/dL - Smoothie with ½ cup berries, protein powder, Greek yogurt, nut butter: spike to 110 mg/dL - Solution: Limit fruit, add protein and fat

**Mistake 4: Oversized portions of everything** - Even a balanced plate can spike if you eat 2-3 servings - Your CGM will show: smaller, balanced meals > large balanced meals - Solution: Use smaller plates, eat slowly, stop at satisfied (not stuffed)

**The Balanced Meal + Portion Control Advantage**:

When you eat balanced meals in appropriate portions: -**Glucose spikes are normal but controlled**:

Post-meal glucose will rise (this is natural and expected), but peaks stay under 130 mg/dL and return to baseline within 90-120 minutes

**Insulin stays low**: Less fat storage, more fat burning between meals

**Hunger decreases**: Protein and fat keep you satisfied for 4-5 hours

**Energy stays high**: No glucose roller coaster, no crashes –

**Cravings disappear**: Stable glucose means no reactive hypoglycemia driving carb cravings

**Weight loss accelerates**: Your body can access stored fat for fuel

**Understanding Normal Post-Meal Glucose Responses:**

**It's completely normal for glucose to spike after eating.** Everyone's glucose rises after a meal, even people with perfect metabolic health. The question is: -

**How high?** Ideally less than 30 mg/dL above your baseline –

**How long?** Should return to within 10 mg/dL of baseline within 90-120 minutes

**Example of a Healthy Response:** - Baseline before meal: 85 mg/dL - Peak 30-60 min after eating: 110 mg/dL (rise of 25 mg/dL) - Back to baseline within 90 minutes: 88 mg/dL - **This is excellent glucose control**

**Example of a Problematic Response:** - Baseline before meal: 90 mg/dL - Peak 45 min after eating: 165 mg/dL (rise of 75 mg/dL) - Still elevated 3 hours later: 115 mg/dL - **This indicates insulin resistance and needs intervention**

Your CGM will teach you which meals create healthy responses, and which don't—then you adjust accordingly.

**Your CGM as Your Personal Portion Guide**:

Generic portion advice doesn't account for YOUR metabolism. Your CGM reveals your unique tolerances:

- Some people can eat 1 cup of rice without spiking
- Others can only handle ¼ cup
- Some tolerate oatmeal well
- Others spike dramatically

**The Protocol**:

1. Start with balanced meals using the formula above
2. Test different portion sizes of carbs while keeping protein, fat, and vegetables constant
3. Find the "sweet spot" where you stay under 130 mg/dL
4. Make that your standard portion
5. You now have personalized portion control based on YOUR body's response

**The Beautiful Result**: You never have to count calories or weigh food obsessively. You simply eat balanced plates with portions that your CGM has shown work for your metabolism. It becomes intuitive.

*3. Exercise: Three Essential Types*

Don't just move—move with purpose across three distinct modalities. Each type of exercise affects your glucose and metabolism differently. Above all choose the one that you're most comfortable with, and don't obsess about it:

**A. Meditation (Mind-Body Exercise)**

**What It Is**: Mindful movement practices that reduce stress and cortisol

**Examples**:

- **Yoga**: focusing on breath and flow

- **Tai Chi**: Gentle, meditative movements

- **Walking Meditation**: Slow, mindful walking in nature

- **Qigong**: Ancient Chinese practice combining breath and movement

**Why It Matters**: Your CGM will show that chronic stress elevates baseline glucose. Meditation practices lower cortisol, which directly improves glucose control and insulin sensitivity.

**Minimum Effective Dose**: 10-15 minutes daily, preferably in the morning or before bed

**B. Stretch (Flexibility and Mobility)**

**What It Is**: Dynamic stretching and mobility work that keeps your body functional and reduces injury risk

**Examples**:

- **Morning stretching routine**: 10 minutes of full-body stretches upon waking - **Foam rolling**: Self-myofascial release for muscle recovery - **Dynamic warm-ups**: Before strength training or walks - **Evening wind-down**

**stretches**: Gentle stretches before bed to improve sleep

**Why It Matters**: Improved mobility means you can exercise more consistently and with better form. Better sleep from evening stretching improves next-day glucose control.

**Minimum Effective Dose**: 10 minutes daily, split between morning and evening

**What It Is**: Dynamic stretching and mobility work that keeps your body functional and reduces injury risk

**C. Strength Training (Muscle Building)**

**What It Is**: Resistance exercise that builds and maintains muscle mass

**Examples**:

- **Bodyweight exercises**: Push-ups, squats, lunges, planks (no equipment needed)

- **Resistance bands**: Portable and effective for all major muscle groups - **Free weights**: Dumbbells or kettlebells for compound movements

- **Gym machines**: Guided resistance training for beginners

**Sample Beginner Routine** (20-30 minutes, 3x per week):

- Squats or goblet squats: 3 sets of 10-12 reps

-Push-ups (modified if needed): 3 sets of 8-10 reps

- Rows (band or dumbbell): 3 sets of 10-12 reps
- Plank holds: 3 sets of 20-30 seconds
- Lunges: 2 sets of 8-10 per leg

**Why It Matters**: Muscle is metabolically active tissue. More muscle means better glucose disposal, higher resting metabolism, and improved insulin sensitivity.

**Minimum Effective Dose**: 20-30 minutes, 2-3 times per week, hitting all major muscle groups

- Plank holds: 3 sets of 20-30 seconds

**The Three-Type Synergy**:

- **Meditation** calms your nervous system and lowers stress-induced glucose spikes
- **Stretching** keeps you mobile so you can exercise consistently
- **Strength training** builds the metabolic machinery that processes glucose efficiently

Together, these three types create a complete exercise program that supports metabolic health from every angle.

*4. Sleep Well*

**What It Means**: 7-9 hours of quality sleep per night, on a consistent schedule

**Non-Negotiable Sleep Practices**:

- Same bedtime and wake time every day (even weekends)
    - No food 3 hours before bed
    - Dark, cool bedroom (65-68°F / 18-20°C)
    - No screens 1 hour before bed
    - No caffeine after 2 PM

**Why It Matters**: Poor sleep consistently increases insulin resistance and raises fasting glucose the following day — research suggests reductions in insulin sensitivity of 25–30% in controlled conditions. Your CGM will show higher baseline glucose and larger spikes after poor sleep, making the connection personal and immediate. Good sleep is the foundation everything else is built on. [Spiegel et al., 1999, The Lancet]

- No food 3 hours before bed
- Dark, cool bedroom (65-68°F / 18-20°C)
- No screens 1 hour before bed

**Examples of Good Sleep Hygiene**:

- **Evening routine**: Dim lights at 8 PM, stretching at 9 PM, reading in bed at 9:30 PM, sleep by 10 PM - **Morning routine**: Wake at 6 AM, get sunlight exposure within 30 minutes to set circadian rhythm

- **Weekend consistency**: If you sleep 10 PM-6 AM on weekdays, maintain the same schedule on weekends

5. *Love Yourself*

**What It Means**: Practice radical self-compassion, speak to yourself with kindness, and release perfectionism

**Non-Negotiable Self-Love Practices**:

- **Mirror work**: Look at yourself daily and say one thing you appreciate
- **Compassionate self-talk**: Speak to yourself as you would to a beloved friend
- **Release comparison**: Your CGM data is yours alone; don't compare to others
- **Celebrate small wins**: Every stable glucose day, every post-meal walks, every kind word to yourself matters
- **Practice forgiveness**: When you spike, when you skip a walk, when you don't sleep well—forgive yourself and continue

**Examples**:

- **When you see a glucose spike**: Instead of "I'm so stupid for eating that," try "My glucose spiked to 155. That's useful information. What can I learn?"

- **When you miss a walk**: Instead of "I'm so lazy and undisciplined," try "I was tired today. Tomorrow I'll walk after breakfast."

- **When progress feels slow**: Instead of "This isn't working," try "My body is healing at its own pace. I'm doing the work."

**Why It Matters**: Chronic self-criticism elevates cortisol, which raises glucose and promotes fat storage. Self-love and stress management directly improve your metabolic health. This isn't just "feel-good" advice—it's metabolically essential.

*6. Track Your Progress (But Don't Obsess)*

**The Minimum**: Wear your CGM, notice patterns, and adjust based on what you learn. You don't need to log every meal or analyze every data point—just pay attention and respond.

**What Good Tracking Looks Like**: - Check your CGM after meals to see the impact - Note which foods keep you stable - Observe how sleep and stress affect your glucose - Adjust your behaviors based on your personal data - Review weekly patterns to identify trends

**What Obsessive Tracking Looks Like (Avoid This)**: - Checking CGM every 5 minutes with anxiety - Panicking over every small spike -

Restricting food to dangerous levels to avoid any glucose elevation - Losing sleep worrying about glucose data - Becoming so rigid you can't enjoy life

**Balance**: Use the CGM as a tool for learning and feedback, not as a judge of your worth.

### The Power of These Six Core Practices

If you wake up tomorrow and implement only these six things—post-meal walks, balanced meals with portion control, three types of exercise, quality sleep, self-love, and mindful CGM tracking—you will transform your metabolic health.

Everything else in this book enhances and optimizes these fundamentals, but these six form the unshakable foundation. Master these first. Make them automatic. Let them become who you are.

Then, when you're ready, layer in the additional strategies and refinements you'll learn in the chapters ahead.

But if you're ever overwhelmed, come back to these six. They're enough.

### What This Book Will Teach You

This book will show you how to harness CGM technology to optimize all four dimensions simultaneously:

- **Metrics**: How to read, interpret, and act on your glucose data
- **Stress**: How to transform your relationship with yourself and food
- **Sleep**: How to use glucose data to optimize your sleep for maximum fat loss
- **Activity**: How to strategically time movement for metabolic transformation

By the end of this journey, you won't just have lost weight—you'll have gained a deep understanding of your unique metabolism and built sustainable habits across all four dimensions that keep the weight off permanently.

This is personalized nutrition in its truest form. Not a celebrity's meal plan or a bestselling diet book, but your body's actual metabolic responses, revealed in unprecedented detail across every dimension that matters.

Let's begin.

> *A note on working with your healthcare team: The approaches in this book — food sequencing, post-meal walking, sleep, and stress management — are designed to work beautifully alongside any care your doctor has recommended, including medication. Think of CGM-guided lifestyle as an additional layer of self-knowledge that makes every other health decision more informed. Please do share what you learn with your physician. The data you gather is genuinely useful to them, and the habits you build here*

*support any treatment plan you are on. →* ***See: A Note on Evidence, Independence, and Medication***

# PART 1: QUICK START GUIDE

## Start Your Transformation TODAY!

**Note:** This Quick Start Guide is designed to get you into action immediately. If you want to dive in right now and start seeing results within 7 days, follow this section first. Then come back and PART 2 of book to understand the "why" behind everything.

**If you prefer to understand the full science first**, skip to Chapter 1 and come back to this guide when you're ready to implement.

–

## Hey there, Future You!

Let's be real: You didn't pick up this guide to read a textbook. You want to lose weight, feel amazing, and understand what the heck is going on with your body. Right?

**Good news:** This is the simplest, most visual guide to weight loss you'll ever read.

**Better news:** It works (and you'll see proof on your phone every day).

**Best news:** No calorie counting. No starvation.

–

## Is This Guide for You?

Check all that apply:

- I want to lose weight but I'm sick of complicated diets
- I hate counting calories (who doesn't?)
- I want to SEE what's happening in my body in real-time
- I'm tired of yo-yo dieting and want something sustainable
- I like visual explanations (charts > walls of text)
- I'm ready to DO something (not just read about it)

**If you checked 3 or more boxes**, keep reading. This is for you.

–

## What You Need to Get Started

### ☐A CGM Device (My New Superpower)

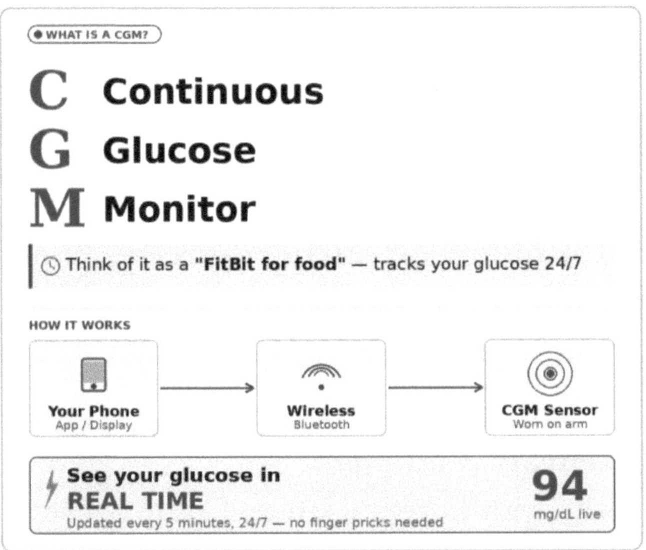


**Where to get one: -**

- Lingo by Abbott (used by the author) – hellolingo.com

For other CGM options available in your region, search "CGM for wellness" or "continuous glucose monitor" in your local search engine. Availability and pricing vary by country.

You may have a different provider in your region.

**How it works:**

1. Stick sensor on your arm (painless, takes 5 seconds)
2. Connect to app on your phone
3. Watch your glucose levels update every few minutes (Don't Obsess)

4. Learn what foods help or hurt you
5. Learn how intentional movement like exercise, or hurt you

## CGM sensor tips

### Sensor falling off during exercise?

- Use adhesive overlay patches or medical tape
- Choose upper arm placement for active lifestyles

### Inaccurate readings?

- Verify with fingerstick test if readings seem wrong
- Contact manufacturer for free replacement if defective
- Trust patterns and trends, not single data points

Occasional sensor issues are normal. Most sensors work perfectly 90-95% of the time.

> The stories below are composite illustrations drawn from common CGM user patterns. They show the range of outcomes that is possible — not a prescription for who this program is for. The author's own journey is the first story; the rest represent typical patterns seen across CGM users. Where a starting health profile falls outside the typical scope of this book (e.g. prediabetes), physician supervision is noted and required.

## SUCCESS STORIES

**My Story: "I Found My Superpower"** *it could be you*

```
BEFORE                  AFTER
______                  _____

Weight: 215 lbs.        Weight: 195 lbs.
Waist: 38"              Waist: 34"
HbA1c: 7.1              HbA1c: 6.2

TIME: 3 months
LOST: 20 lbs.
```

**What I did:** - Walked 90 min/day total (after major meal) – Took balanced meal every time,

increased protein, included healthy fat and cut down carbs not did not remove it altogether. Fixed my sleep (7-8 hours) - Checked CGM religiously
**My secret:** "The CGM was my superpower. I could SEE what foods were sabotaging me and how exercise affected the readings. Once I saw it, I couldn't unsee it. Game changer!"

**Example Story: "I Stopped Starving Myself"** *it could be you*

```
BEFORE                      AFTER
______                      _____

Age: 38                     Age: 38
Weight: 180 lbs.             Weight: 155 lbs
Eating: 1200 cal/day        Eating: 1800 cal
Mood: Miserable             Mood: Fantastic
Cravings: Constant          Cravings: None
Energy: Exhausted           Energy: Amazing


TIME: 4 months
LOST: 25 lbs (eating MORE food!)
```

**What changed:** - Stopped calorie counting - Focused on glucose-stable foods - Ate when hungry (but right foods) - 30-min walks after meals - Got serious about sleep

**The secret:** "I was eating MORE food but losing weight because my glucose was stable. No more crashes. No more cravings. It felt like magic, but it was just science!"

**Example Story: "My Body, My Rules" IT COULD BE YOU**

*Note: This composite example includes a starting A1C of 6.2% (prediabetes range). As stated in the Medical*

*Disclaimer, individuals with prediabetes must work with their healthcare team before using a CGM independently. This story illustrates metabolic improvement patterns; it does not represent a typical starting profile for this program. If your A1C is 5.7% or above, please consult your physician before beginning.*

```
BEFORE                        AFTER
________                        _____

Age: 52                         Age: 52
Weight: 240 lbs.                Weight: 205 lbs
A1C: 6.2 (prediabetic) A1C: 5.4 (normal)
Medications: 2                   Medications: 0
Doctor visits: Monthly           Doctor: Amazed

 TIME: 6 months
 LOST: 35 lbs.+ reversed prediabetes!
```

**What changed:** - Used CGM to find trigger foods - Discovered white rice was fine, oatmeal was terrible (opposite of what he expected!) - Walked religiously - Strength trained consistently - Became a morning person (better sleep)

**The secret:** "Everyone's different. The CGM showed me MY body's rules, not some generic diet rules. That's why it worked!"

Throughout this book you will see weight loss described as four interconnected dimensions: real-time metrics, movement, sleep, and stress management. Those four dimensions explain the 'why' — the metabolic forces that drive fat storage and fat burning.

The six rules below are the 'how' — the practical daily habits that address all four dimensions simultaneously. Rules 1–3 cover metrics and movement. Rule 4 covers sleep. Rule 5 (Love Yourself) is the actionable expression of stress management and self-compassion. Rule 6 (Track Your CGM) is how you apply the real-time metrics dimension day to day.

**A note on the framework:**

***Four dimensions, six daily practices — one goal.***

## The 6 Golden Rules (THIS IS ALL YOU NEED)

Let me make this crystal clear: **Many people who consistently follow these 6 rules report meaningful improvements in weight and energy within the first 30 days. Individual results vary based on starting health, adherence, and metabolism.**

No ifs, ands, or buts. Let's go!

*Individual results vary based on metabolism, starting health, and adherence. This program is not a substitute for medical advice. Consult your healthcare provider before starting any new diet or exercise program. If you have diabetes, prediabetes, or any medical condition, additional guidance is required. See full disclaimer on copyright page.*

-

## RULE #1: Walk 30 Minutes After EVERY Meal

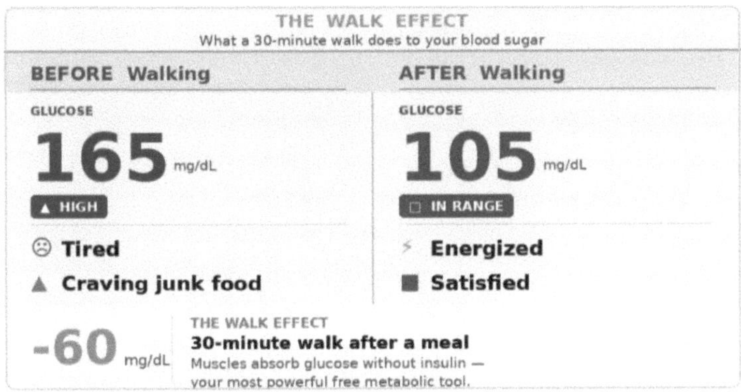


Let me make this crystal clear:

**Why this works:**

When you eat, your glucose goes up. Your body releases insulin to bring it down. While insulin is high, **fat burning is significantly suppressed**. Elevated insulin strongly inhibits fat oxidation, keeping your body in energy-storage mode rather than fat-burning mode.

Walking after meals: -

Lowers glucose faster ⚡ -

Meaningfully reduces insulin exposure –

Unlocks fat-burning mode –

Takes only 30 minutes

**My Daily Walking Schedule or you may choose a different activity that makes you move:**

Lowers glucose faster ⚡ -

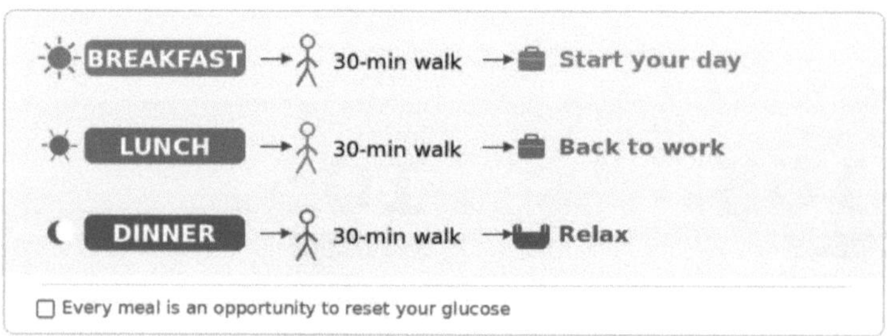


`TOTAL: 90 minutes walking per day. (Yes, it's worth it. Yes, you have time. I'll prove it.)`

**PRO TIPS:**

**Make it fun:** - Listen to podcasts - Call a friend - Audio books - Music playlist

**Make it social:** - Walk with spouse/partner - Family walk after dinner - Walking meetings at work - Join a walking group

**"I don't have time!" → YES, YOU DO:**

Think about it: - Scrolling social media: 2+ hours/day - Watching TV: 3+ hours/day - **Walking for your health: 90 minutes/day**

You're not too busy. You're just not prioritizing it (yet).

**START SMALL IF YOU MUST:**

```
Week 1: 10 minutes after each meal = 30 min/day
Week 2: 15 minutes after each meal = 45 min/day
Week 3: 20 minutes after each meal = 60 min/day
Week 4: 25 minutes after each meal = 75 min/day
Week 5+: 30 minutes after each meal = 90 min/day []
```

## A Note on Walking Alternatives

I lost my 20 pounds by walking 90 minutes in a day. It worked perfectly for me—I had the flexibility in my schedule, the weather was generally cooperative, and I enjoyed being outside.

But I know not everyone has those advantages.

Maybe you live somewhere with harsh winters. Maybe you have a knee injury. Maybe you work in an office were disappearing for 30 minutes after lunch isn't realistic. Maybe you're a parent with young kids who can't leave them to go walk.

**Here's the truth:** The goal isn't walking. The goal is lowering your glucose after meals.

Walking worked for me because it's a simple, accessible way to use muscle movement to burn glucose. But it's not the ONLY way.

In Appendix B, I'll share alternatives that achieve the same glucose-lowering effect—some are even MORE effective than walking! Whether you need indoor options, have mobility limitations, live in extreme climates, or simply prefer other activities, there's a solution that will work for you.

## RULE #2: Build the Perfect Plate

### The Glucose-Stable Plate Formula:

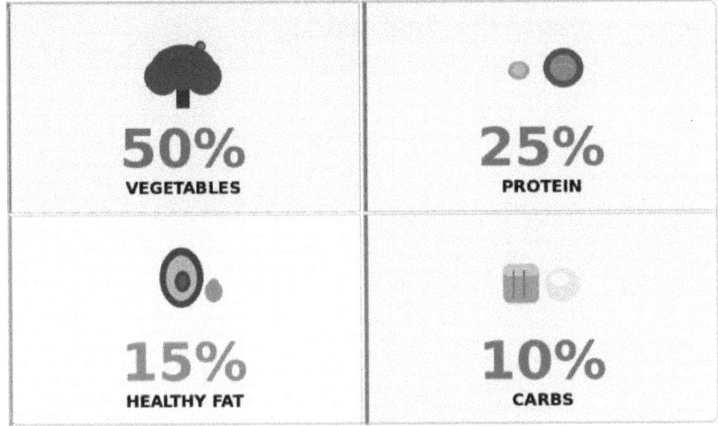


### START SMALL IF YOU MUST:

### THE HAND METHOD (Never Measure Again):

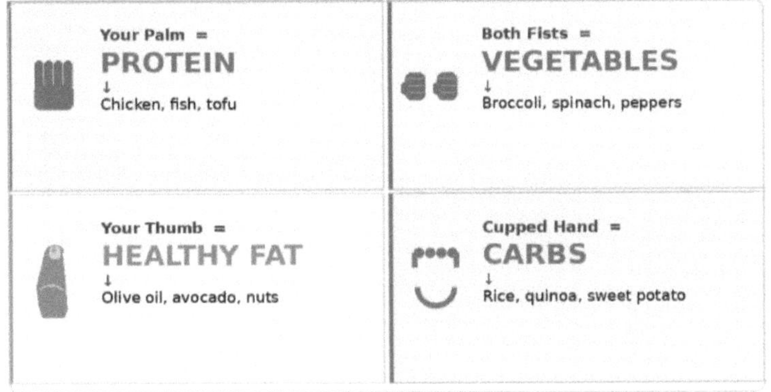

YOUR PLATE = 50% non-starchy vegetables · 25% protein · 25% healthy fat + a small portion of complex carbs (within that final quarter)

Where do carbohydrates fit? Carbs share the final 25% quarter with your healthy fat — they are not a separate allocation. Think of it as: a fist-sized serving of complex carbs (sweet potato, quinoa, legumes, or whole grain) alongside your fat source (avocado, olive oil, or a small handful of nuts). Your CGM will show you exactly how much carbohydrate your metabolism can handle in that quarter before a problematic spike occurs — that is your personal carb tolerance, and it is unique to you.

**THE HAND METHOD (Never Measure Again):**

**REAL PLATE EXAMPLES:**

The foods shown in this guide are examples to teach the concept. YOU get to choose:

YOUR favorite vegetables (any kind!)

YOUR favorite protein sources

YOUR favorite healthy fats

YOUR favorite carbohydrate sources

The magic is in the PROPORTIONS (50% veggies, 25% protein, 25% fats + carbs), not the specific foods.

**Examples:**

• Hate broccoli? Use spinach, bok choy, or any greens you enjoy!

• Don't eat meat? Use tofu, beans, lentils, or plant-based proteins!

• Allergic to avocado? Use olive oil, nuts, seeds, or coconut!

• Following keto? Skip or minimize the carbs!

• Vegetarian or vegan? Perfect—plenty of plant-based options!

**Cultural Note:**

The food examples in this book reflect common Western ingredients, but the glucose-stable plate formula works with ANY cuisine:

• Indian cuisine? Dal, vegetables, and ghee work perfectly!

• Asian diet? Rice with stir-fried veggies and protein fits the formula!

• Mediterranean? Olive oil, fish, and vegetables are ideal!

• Middle Eastern? Hummus, falafel, and abundant vegetables work great!

• Latin American? Beans, avocado, and vegetables are perfect!

• African? Traditional stews with vegetables and protein fit beautifully!

The 50/25/25 ratio is universal—the specific foods are YOUR choice based on your culture, preferences, and what's available to you.

**Make it YOURS.**

**Breakfast Winner:**

**Note:** Examples shown. Choose your own preferred foods from each category. The ratios matter. Customize to your taste, dietary needs, and preferences.

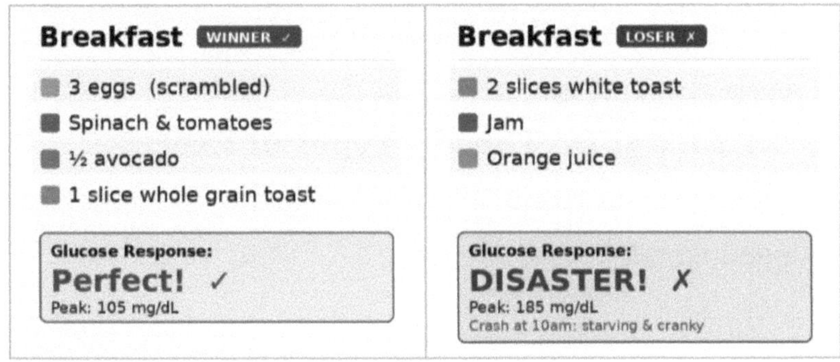


**THE FOOD SEQUENCING HACK:**

Want to reduce glucose spikes by 40%? Eat in this order: [Imai et al., 2014, Diabetes Care; Shukla et al., 2017, Diabetes Care, 38(7), e98–e99. [PubMed: 25931478]]

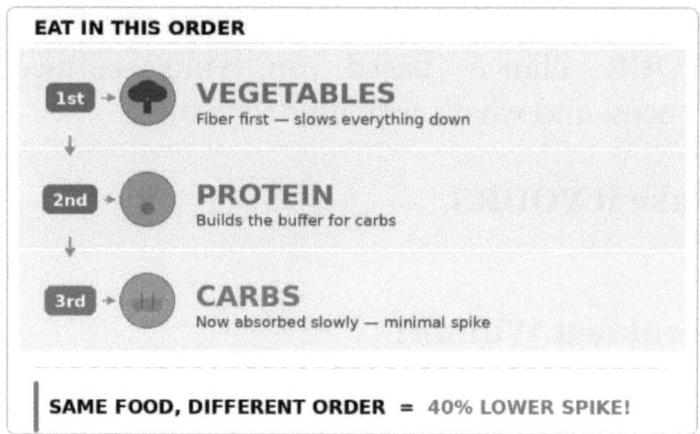


**Note:** Examples shown. Choose your own preferred foods from each category. The ratios matter. Customize to your taste, dietary needs, and preferences.

**Why this works:** Fiber and protein slow down carb absorption!

**RULE #3: Do These 3 Types of Exercise**

Most people think exercise = cardio. Wrong! You need variety.

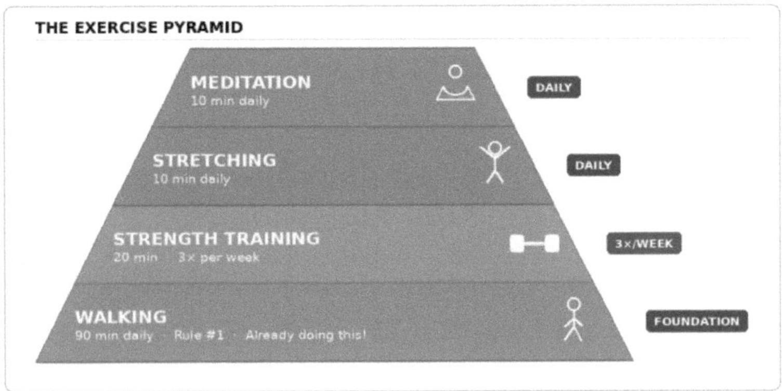


## TYPE 1: MEDITATION/MIND-BODY (Stress Reduction)

**Why:** Stress = Cortisol ↑ = Glucose ↑ = Fat Storage ↑

**What to do (pick one or something better you might have):** -

Yoga (10-15 min)
Tai Chi
Walking meditation
Deep breathing exercises

**When:** Every morning before breakfast

**SIMPLE 10-MINUTE MORNING ROUTINE:**

```
1. Wake up
2. Drink water
3. 5 minutes stretching
4. 5 minutes deep breathing
```

5. Eat breakfast
6. Walk 30 minutes

**TYPE 2: STRETCHING (Flexibility & Recovery)**

**Why:** Prevents injury, improves sleep, lowers stress

**What to do:** - Morning: 5 min full body stretch - Evening: 5 min wind-down stretch

**When:** Morning and before bed

**TYPE 3: STRENGTH TRAINING (Build Muscle = Burn Fat)**

**Why: More muscle = higher metabolism 24/7**

**The "Lazy Person's" Strength Routine:**

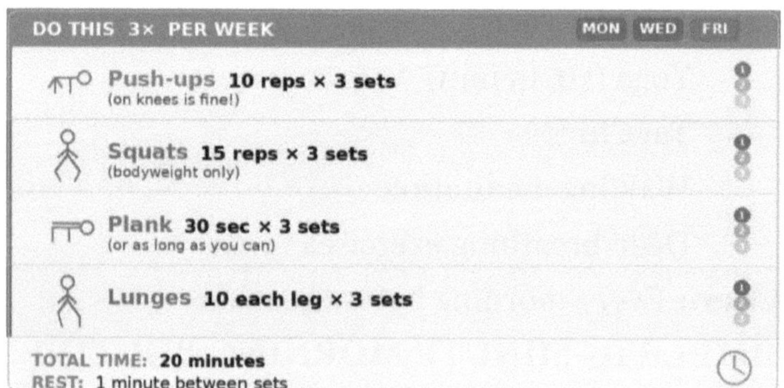


**What to do:** - Morning: 5 min full body stretch - Evening: 5 min wind-down stretch

**WHAT HAPPENS TO YOUR GLUCOSE:**

```
During Strength Training:
  ↗ Glucose goes UP (normal!)

24-48 Hours AFTER:
  ↘ Glucose sensitivity IMPROVES
   Fat burning INCREASES
   Muscle mass GROWS
  This is why you do it!
```

## RULE #4: Sleep Like Your Life Depends on It (It Does)

## The Sleep-Glucose Connection:

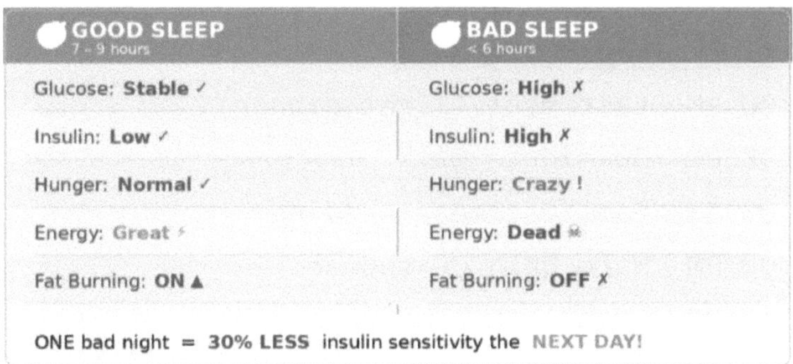

| GOOD SLEEP<br>7 - 9 hours | BAD SLEEP<br>< 6 hours |
|---|---|
| Glucose: **Stable** ✓ | Glucose: **High** ✗ |
| Insulin: **Low** ✓ | Insulin: **High** ✗ |
| Hunger: **Normal** ✓ | Hunger: **Crazy** ! |
| Energy: **Great** ⚡ | Energy: **Dead** ☠ |
| Fat Burning: **ON** ▲ | Fat Burning: **OFF** ✗ |

ONE bad night = **30% LESS** insulin sensitivity the NEXT DAY!

## WHAT HAPPENS TO YOUR GLUCOSE:

## THE 5 SLEEP COMMANDMENTS:

```
1️⃣ SAME TIME EVERY DAY
   Bed: 10 PM | Wake: 6 AM
   (Even weekends!)

2️⃣ NO FOOD 3 HOURS BEFORE BED
   Last meal: 7 PM | Bed: 10 PM
```

3️⃣NO SCREENS 1 HOUR BEFORE BED

Phone down: 9 PM | Bed: 10 PM

4️⃣NO CAFFEINE AFTER 2 PM

Coffee cutoff: 2 PM →

5️⃣COOL, DARK ROOM

Temp: 65-68°F (18-20°C)

Blackout curtains ON

**YOUR PERFECT EVENING ROUTINE – remember we're not seeking perfection but simply weight loss:**

7:00 PM Last meal (light dinner)

7:30 PM 30-minute walk

8:00 PM Family time / Reading

9:00 PM Warm bath or shower

9:15 PM Light stretching (5 min)

9:30 PM Phone in another room

9:45 PM Read a book (physical, not tablet!)

10:00 PM Lights out

6:00 AM Wake up refreshed!

**SLEEP HACKS:**

White noise machine or fan

Eye mask if needed

Chamomile tea at 8 PM

Journal for 5 min (brain dump worries)

## RULE #5: Love Yourself (This Is Non-Negotiable)

## The Mind-Body Connection:

| NEGATIVE SELF-TALK | POSITIVE SELF-TALK |
|---|---|
| Stress | Stress |
| ↓ | ↓ |
| Cortisol | Cortisol |
| ↓ | ↓ |
| Glucose | Glucose |
| ↓ | ↓ |
| Fat Storage | Fat Burning |

Your THOUGHTS affect your WEIGHT!

Your THOUGHTS affect your WEIGHT!

## DAILY MIRROR WORK (Do This Every Morning):

Stand in front of mirror.

Look yourself in the eye.

Say out loud:

[] "I am getting healthier every day"

[] "I am worthy of feeling good"

[] "I am capable of change"

[] "I love and accept myself"

[] "Progress, not perfection"

Sounds cheesy? DO IT ANYWAY.

It works. Trust me.

**STOP THESE TOXIC THOUGHTS:**

"I'm so fat and disgusting"

[] "I'm working on my health"

"I have no willpower"

[] "I'm building new habits"

"I'll never lose this weight"

[] "I'm making progress every day"

"I ruined everything with one meal"

[] "One meal doesn't define my journey"

**THE BAD DAY PROTOCOL:**

Had a rough day? Ate poorly? Skipped your walk?

STOP. BREATHE. DO THIS:

1. Forgive yourself (seriously, RIGHT NOW)
2. Don't spiral into guilt
3. Don't "start over Monday"
4. Just get back on track NEXT MEAL
5. One bad meal ≠ One bad day
6. One bad day ≠ One bad week

YOU'RE HUMAN. IT'S OKAY.

## RULE #6: Check Your CGM (But Don't Obsess)

## Good Tracking vs. Bad Tracking:

| ☑ GOOD TRACKING | ☒ BAD TRACKING |
|---|---|
| • Check 3-4× daily | – Check every 5 min |
| • Look after meals | – Panic at every number |
| • Learn patterns | – Stress about perfection |
| • Adjust based on data | – Let it control you |
| • Feel empowered | – Feel anxious |

◎ CGM = Learning tool, NOT a judge!

YOU'RE HUMAN. IT'S OKAY.

## WHEN TO CHECK YOUR CGM:

```
 Morning: Fasting glucose
   Target: 70-90 mg/dL

 1 hour after breakfast
   Target: Return toward baseline

 1 hour after lunch
   Target: Return toward baseline

 1 hour after dinner
   Target: Return toward baseline
```

```
Before bed
   Target: 80-100 mg/dL
```

## UNDERSTANDING YOUR NUMBERS:

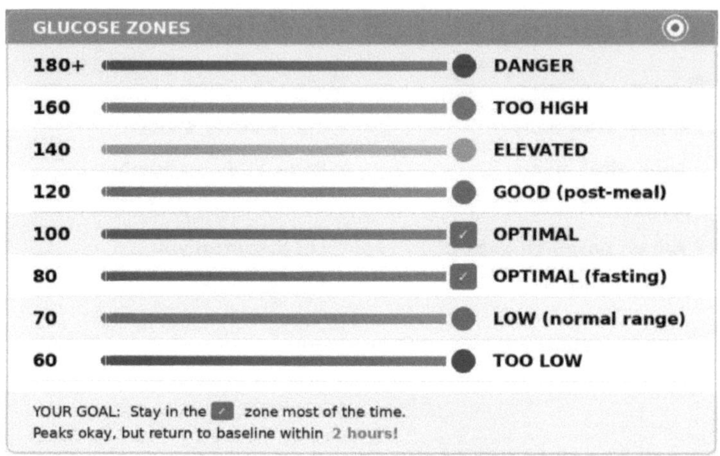


## Good Tracking vs. Bad Tracking:

## THE 2-HOUR RULE:

```
Whatever you eat, your glucose should:

  1. Peak within 1 hour ⏱

  2. Return to baseline within 2 hours ⏱⏱

Example:
  8:00 AM - Eat breakfast (glucose: 85)
  9:00 AM - Peak (glucose: 115) ← +30 rise
  10:00 AM - Back to baseline (glucose: 88)
[]
```

```
If it takes 3+ hours to return = problem!
```

# YOUR 30-DAY TRANSFORMATION PLAN

## WEEK 1-2: LEARN MODE

**Goal:** Understand your body without changing too much

### YOUR FOOD EXPERIMENTS:

Test these foods or the ones you normally take with some variations and watch your CGM – data doesn't lie:

**Note:** Examples shown. Choose your own preferred foods from each category. The ratios matter, not the specific foods listed. Customize to your taste, dietary needs, and preferences.

```
WEEK 1-2 CHECKLIST

  [] Got CGM and connected to app
  [] Eating normally (for now)
  [] Walking after meals
  [] Checking glucose 4x daily
  [] Taking notes on what you observe

  WHAT YOU'LL LEARN:
   Which foods spike your glucose
   Which foods keep you stable
```

```
How much walking helps
Your unique metabolic patterns
```

```
TEST #1: White rice vs. Brown rice
   Monday lunch: White rice
   Tuesday lunch: Brown rice
  Which one keeps you more stable?

TEST #2: Toast vs. Eggs
   Wednesday breakfast: Toast
   Thursday breakfast: Eggs
  Which gives better energy?

TEST #3: Apple vs. Candy bar
   Friday snack: Apple
   Saturday snack: Candy
  See the difference!

TEST #4: Juice vs. Whole fruit
   Sunday: Orange juice
   Monday: Whole orange
  Massive difference!
```

**KEEP A SIMPLE LOG:** Of course! your CGM app keeps history, but you may have to input the meal entry

```
Date:

Meal: Breakfast
```

```
Food:
Time eaten:
Glucose before:
Glucose 1hr after:
How I feel:

Notes: ____________________
```

## WEEK 3-4: CHANGE MODE

**Goal:** Apply what you learned, start making swaps

```
WEEK 3-4 CHECKLIST

[] Stop eating foods that spike you
[] Eat more foods that keep you stable
[] Build the perfect plate (Rule #2)
[] Walk after ALL meals (no excuses)
[] Start strength training (3x week)
[] Fix your sleep routine

WHAT YOU'LL SEE:
⚡ More stable energy
 Less hunger/cravings
 Glucose staying in optimal zone
 Better mood
```

## THE SMART SWAP STRATEGY:

| INSTEAD OF THIS... | | EAT THIS INSTEAD |
|---|---|---|
| White bread | → | Whole grain |
| Sugary cereal | → | Eggs |
| Juice | → | Whole fruit |
| Pasta | → | Zoodles |
| Chips | → | Nuts |
| Soda | → | Sparkling water |
| Candy | → | Berries |
| Ice cream | → | Greek yogurt |
| SAME SATISFACTION, BETTER GLUCOSE! | | |

## WEEK 5-6: HABIT MODE

**Goal:** Make it automatic, build your routine

```
WEEK 5-6 CHECKLIST

[] 6 rules are becoming automatic
[] Walking feels natural
[] Healthy eating is easier
[] Sleep routine is solid
[] You know your trigger foods
[] Family/friends are supportive

WHAT YOU'LL FEEL:
 Stronger and more confident
⚡ Consistent energy all day
 Better sleep quality
```

In control of your choices

## MILESTONE CHECK:

By end of Week 6, you should have:

[] Lost 5-10 lbs (2-4 kg)

[] Better fitting clothes

[] More energy

[] Fewer cravings

[] Stable mood

[] Better sleep

[] Confident in your routine

IF NOT? Review the 6 rules.

Which ones are you skipping?

## WEEK 7-8+: RESULTS MODE

**Goal:** See the transformation, keep momentum

```
WEEK 7-8+ CHECKLIST

[] Continue 6 rules daily
[] Track weight weekly (not daily!)
[] Celebrate non-scale victories
[] Help others (share what you learned)
[] Plan for long-term success

WHAT YOU'LL ACHIEVE:
 10-15 lbs lost (4-7 kg)
 Clothes fit better
 People notice your transformation
 You feel like a new person
```

# VISUAL TRANSFORMATION TIMELINE

VISUAL TRANSFORMATION TIMELINE
MONTH 1
MONTH 2
MONTH 3
MONTH 6
Starting weight
-5 lbs.
Better energy
Getting momentum
-10 lbs.
Much more energy
Confident habit
-15 lbs.
Clothes size down
New You
-20-30 lbs.
Better health
People asking your secret!
THE TRANSFORMATION JOURNEY

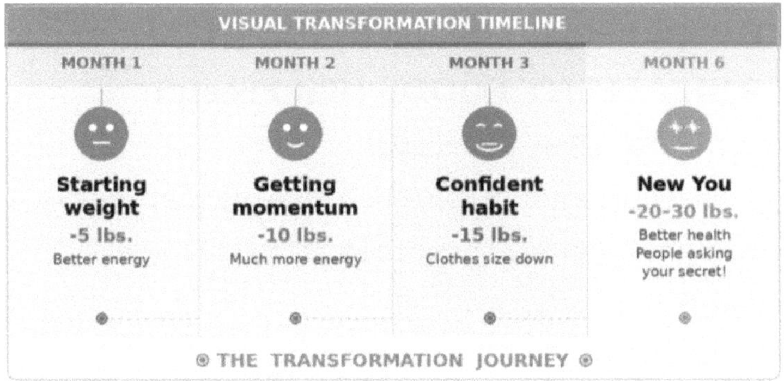

## THE SUGGESTED FOOD GUIDE – best to consult your nutritionist, see your personal data on the CGM

### GREEN LIGHT FOODS (Eat Freely)

```
VEGETABLES (Non-Starchy)
├── Leafy greens  (spinach, kale, lettuce)
├── Cruciferous  (broccoli, cauliflower,
cabbage)
├── Peppers  (bell peppers, jalapeños)
├── Cucumbers
├── Tomatoes
├── Zucchini
├── Mushrooms
├── Asparagus
└── Green beans

PROTEINS
├── Fish  (salmon, tuna, cod)
├── Chicken
├── Turkey
├── Eggs
├── Greek yogurt (plain)
├── Cottage cheese
└── Tofu

HEALTHY FATS
├── Avocado
```

```
├── Olive oil
├── Nuts (almonds, walnuts)
├── Seeds (chia, flax)
└── Coconut oil
```

## YELLOW LIGHT FOODS (Eat Moderately)

```
COMPLEX CARBS (Small portions)
├── Brown rice (½ cup max)
├── Quinoa
├── Sweet potato (½ medium)
├── Oats (steel-cut, ½ cup)
└── Whole grain bread (1 slice)

FRUITS (Lower sugar)
├── Berries (best choice!)
├── Apples (with skin)
├── Pears
├── Grapefruit
└── Oranges (whole, not juice!)

DAIRY
├── Cheese (small amounts)
└── Milk (limit to ½ cup)
```

## RED LIGHT FOODS (Avoid or Rare Treats)

```
AVOID THESE (At least for first 30 days)
├── Candy
├── Cookies
├── Cake
├── Ice cream
```

```
Check CGM – Working goal: <130 mg/dL post-
meal; optimal aim: <120 mg/dL (see Chapter
4 for full guide)
```

```
├── Soda
├── Juice  (even "healthy" ones!)
├── White bread
├── White rice
├── Pasta  (white)
├── Pizza  (regular crust)
├── Chips
├── Fries
├── Donuts
└── Sugary cereals

YOUR CGM WILL THANK YOU!
```

# SUGGESTED DAILY SCHEDULE TEMPLATE

## PERFECT MORNING ROUTINE

```
6:00 AM    Wake up
          Drink 16 oz water


6:15 AM    10-min meditation/stretching


6:30 AM    Breakfast
         Example:
         - 3 scrambled eggs
```

- Sautéed spinach
- ½ avocado
- 1 slice whole grain toast

7:00 AM 30-minute brisk walk

7:45 AM Check CGM
Target: <120 mg/dL

8:00 AM Start your day!

**PERFECT AFTERNOON ROUTINE**

12:00 PM Lunch
Example:
- Grilled chicken breast
- Large salad
- Olive oil dressing
- ½ cup brown rice

12:30 PM 30-minute walk
(Walking meeting?)

1:15 PM Check CGM
Target: <120 mg/dL

1:30 PM Back to productive work

3:00 PM Hydration check

(16 oz water)

3:30 PM Smart snack (if needed)
- Handful of almonds
- OR apple with almond butter
- OR Greek yogurt

**PERFECT EVENING ROUTINE**

6:00 PM Dinner (early!)
Example:
- Baked salmon
- Steamed broccoli
- Side salad
- Small sweet potato

6:30 PM 30-minute walk
(Family time!)

7:30 PM Check CGM
Target: <120 mg/dL

8:00 PM Kitchen closed!
(No more food)

8:30 PM Relaxation time
- Read
- Light stretching
- Family time

```
9:00 PM    Warm shower

9:30 PM    Phone in another room

9:45 PM    Read physical book

10:00 PM   Lights out

           Magic happens while you sleep!
```

## THE 20-MINUTE WORKOUT

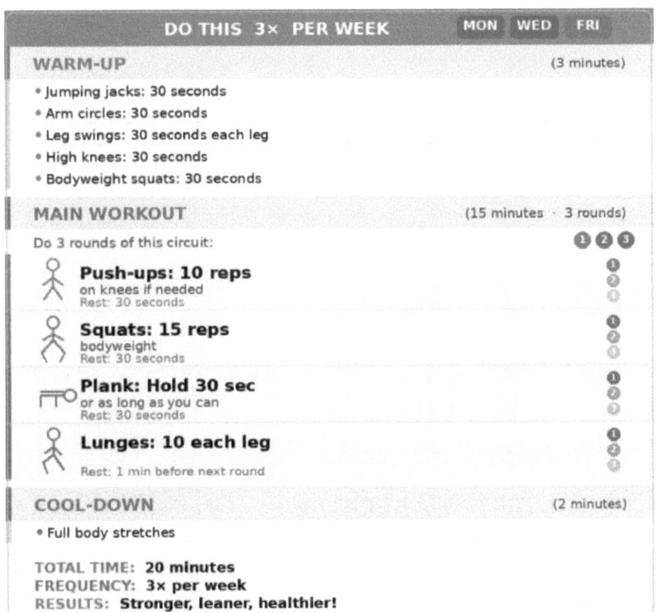

## PROGRESSION PLAN:

```
6:00 PM    Dinner (early!)
             Example:
          - Baked salmon
          - Steamed broccoli
          - Side salad
          - Small sweet potato

6:30 PM    30-minute walk (Family time!)

7:30 PM    Check CGM
          Target: <120 mg/dL

8:00 PM    Kitchen closed!
          (No more food)

8:30 PM    Relaxation time
          - Read
          - Light stretching
          - Family time

9:00 PM    Warm shower

9:30 PM    Phone in another room
```

```
9:45 PM    Read physical book

10:00 PM   Lights out

           Magic happens while you sleep!

_
```

# TROUBLESHOOTING GUIDE

## "My glucose is still spiking!"

```
  POSSIBLE CAUSES:


   Portions too large
     → Solution: Use hand method, eat les
s


   Not walking after meals
     → Solution: Set phone alarms

   Eating carbs first
     → Solution: Veggies → Protein → Carb
s


   Hidden sugars in "healthy" foods
     → Solution: Read labels, check CGM

   Poor sleep last night
     → Solution: Fix sleep tonight!

   High stress
     → Solution: Meditation, deep breathi
ng
```

## "I'm not losing weight!"

```
CHECK THESE:

□ Are you REALLY walking 90 min/day?
  (Be honest!)

□ Are your portions small?
  (Use measuring cups for a week)

□ Are you eating after 7 PM?
  (Kitchen closed = kitchen closed!)

□ Are you sleeping 7-9 hours?
  (Track it!)

□ Are you strength training?
  (Muscle = metabolism!)

□ Are you stressed/not sleeping well?
  (Cortisol blocks weight loss)

□ How long have you been trying?
  (Give it 4 weeks minimum!)
```

**Remember:** The scale is a liar sometimes. Check these instead:

- How do your clothes fit?
- How's your energy? ⚡
- How's your sleep?
- What does the mirror show?

**"I had a bad day/weekend!"**

-

**"I don't have time for 90 minutes of walking!"**

```
REALLY? Let's do the math:

 Time you spend per day:
   - Scrolling social media: 2-3 hours
   - Watching TV: 3-4 hours
   - YouTube/Netflix: 1-2 hours
   ──────────────────────────────
   TOTAL: 6-9 hours on screens

vs.

 Time for your health:
   - Walking: 90 minutes (1.5 hours)

You have time.
You're just not prioritizing it.
```

SOLUTIONS:

[] Walk while listening to podcasts

[] Walk during phone calls

[] Walk during lunch break

[] Walk with family after dinner

[] Wake up 30 min earlier

WHERE THERE'S A WILL, THERE'S A WALK! ♂

```
- STOP RIGHT THERE!

  One bad meal ≠ Failure
  One bad day ≠ Start over Monday
  One bad weekend ≠ All progress lost

  DO THIS INSTEAD:
  1. Forgive yourself (right now!)
  2. Don't spiral into guilt
  3. Get back on track NEXT MEAL
  4. Go for a walk (seriously, now!)
  5. Remember why you started

  YOU'RE HUMAN. YOU GOT THIS!
```

# SUGGESTED YOUR QUICK REFERENCE CHECKLIST

## DAILY CHECKLIST (Print this!)

## SUGGESTED WEEKLY CHECKLIST

WEEKLY REVIEW

□ Weigh yourself (Sunday AM, same time)

□ Take progress photos (same pose/light)

□ Measure waist

□ 3 strength training sessions done

□ Walked 90 min/day for 6-7 days

□ Slept 7-9 hours for 5-7 nights

□ No late-night eating

□ Reviewed CGM patterns

□ Planned next week's meals

□ Celebrated wins (even small ones!)

WEEKLY GOALS:

This week I will: ________________

Last week I learned: ______________

- DAILY MUST-DO's

MORNING:

□ Wake same time (_____ AM)

□ 10-min meditation/stretch

□ Healthy breakfast (50% veggies!)

□ 30-min walk after breakfast

□ Check CGM

AFTERNOON:

□ Healthy lunch (balanced plate)

□ 30-min walk after lunch

□ Check CGM

□ Drink water (64 oz total today)

EVENING:

□ Early dinner (before 7 PM)

□ 30-min walk after dinner

□ Check CGM

□ Kitchen closed at 8 PM

□ Phone away at 9 PM

□ Bed by 10 PM

BONUS:

□ Positive self-talk

□ Gratitude journal (3 things)

□ Helped someone today

# KEY TAKEAWAYS

## THE BIG IDEAS

**5 PRINCIPLES OF EFFORTLESS WEIGHT LOSS**

**#1**

**YOUR GLUCOSE CONTROLS YOUR WEIGHT**

High glucose → High insulin → Fat storage
Stable glucose → Low insulin → Fat burning

**It's that simple.**

**#2**

**WALKING IS YOUR SECRET WEAPON**

30 min after each meal = −50% insulin
That's 90 min/day of fat-burning magic

**Non-negotiable.**

**#3**

**YOU ARE UNIQUE**

Your body responds differently than mine
Your CGM shows YOUR truth
Stop following generic diet advice

**Trust YOUR data.**

**#4**

**SLEEP IS NOT OPTIONAL**

Bad sleep = 30% worse glucose control
7-9 hours = Your metabolism's best friend

**Prioritize it.**

**#5**

**LOVE YOURSELF THROUGH THE PROCESS**

Stress → Cortisol → High glucose → Fat
Self-compassion → Calm → Stable glucose

**Be kind to yourself.**

## SUGGESTED WEEKLY CHECKLIST

# YOUR NEXT STEPS

## RIGHT NOW (Next 5 Minutes)

1. □ Order your CGM (pick a provider, do it NOW)
2. □ Download this guide to your phone
3. □ Set 3 daily alarms:
- Breakfast walk (your time + 30 min)
- Lunch walk (your time + 30 min)
- Dinner walk (your time + 30 min)
4. □ Clear junk food from kitchen
5. □ Text 3 people: "I'm starting a health journey.
   I need your support!"

-

## TODAY (Before Bed)

1. □ Plan tomorrow's meals (write them down)
2. □ Prep breakfast ingredients
3. □ Set out workout clothes
4. □ Set bedtime alarm for 9:30 PM
5. □ Read this guide one more time
6. □ Visualize success (1 minute)
7. □ Get 7-9 hours sleep (seriously!)

## THIS WEEK (Days 1-7)

1. □ CGM arrives → Install → Connect app
2. □ Follow 6 rules every single day
3. □ Track everything (food, walks, sleep)

```
4. □ Take "before" photos (you'll thank me
later)
5. □ Measure: weight, waist, how you feel
6. □ Join online community for support
7. □ Review and adjust
```

## FINAL PEP TALK

Hey, you made it to the end! That alone puts you ahead of 90% of people who just "want to lose weight someday."

Here's the truth: **This is simple, but it's not easy.**

Simple = 6 clear rules

Not easy = Changing habits takes effort

**But you know what's harder?** - Feeling uncomfortable in your body every day - Having no energy to play with your kids - Avoiding photos because you hate how you look - Worrying about your health as you age

**That's harder.**

So yes, walking 90 minutes a day is work.

Yes, preparing healthy meals takes time.

Yes, going to bed early feels like you're missing out.

**But you're not missing out. You're investing in yourself.**

And 30 days from now, when you've lost 10 pounds, have more energy than you've had in years, and people are asking "what's your secret?" ...

You'll know it was worth it.

## ONE LAST THING

This quick-start guide gives you everything you need to get started and see results. But if you want the deep dive — all the science, advanced strategies, troubleshooting, and complete protocols — read the complete guide:

And 30 days from now, when you've lost 10 pounds, have more energy than you've had in years, and people are asking "what's your secret?" ...

You'll know it was worth it.

-

```
    YOUR TRANSFORMATION STARTS NOW

Not Monday. Not after the holidays.
Not when you're "ready."

NOW.

You've got this!
```

**Go get your CGM. Start tomorrow. Change your life. You deserve to feel amazing.**

_**You deserve to feel amazing.**

**P.S.** When you hit your first big milestone, share it! POST on social media.

https://www.facebook.com/profile.php?id=61581317054546

I want to celebrate with you!

_

# PART 2: THE SCIENCE

## Deep Dive into The Science and Strategy

Now that you have your Quick Start action plan, let's dive deep into understanding exactly WHY these strategies work, the science behind glucose control, and how to customize everything for your unique body.

.

# Chapter 1: Understanding Continuous Glucose Monitors

I still remember the moment the app connected and that little line appeared on my phone screen — a quiet, steady graph of my own blood sugar, updating every few minutes. I had no idea what I was looking at. I just knew something had changed: for the first time in my life, my body wasn't a black box anymore. This chapter gives you the foundation to understand what that device on your arm is measuring, and why it matters so much more than the number on your bathroom scale.

## What Is a CGM?

A Continuous Glucose Monitor is a small wearable device, typically about the size of a quarter, that adheres to the back of your upper arm or abdomen. It contains a tiny sensor that sits just beneath your skin, measuring glucose levels in your interstitial fluid (the fluid between your cells) every few minutes, 24 hours a day.

The device wirelessly transmits this data to your smartphone, where you can view your glucose levels in real-time and see patterns throughout the day and night. Most CGMs need to be replaced every 10-14 days.

### CGMs Beyond Diabetes

While CGMs were developed for diabetes management, they're increasingly being used by people without diabetes who want to optimize their health and lose weight.

These services typically combine the CGM hardware with apps that help interpret your data and provide personalized recommendations.

### How CGMs Work

The sensor measures glucose by detecting the chemical reaction between glucose and an enzyme (glucose oxidase) on the sensor filament. This creates a small electrical current proportional to the glucose concentration, which is converted into a glucose reading.

It's important to note that CGM readings can lag blood glucose by 5-15 minutes since they measure interstitial fluid rather than blood directly. For weight loss purposes, this delay is negligible and doesn't affect the insights you'll gain.

## Chapter 2: The Glucose-Weight Connection

Before I put on the CGM, I thought weight loss was simple arithmetic — eat less, move more, suffer enough. What the data showed me in the first week demolished that idea completely. The same meal I'd been eating for years was triggering a cascade of hormonal events that made fat burning almost impossible, and I had no idea it was happening. Understanding this connection changed everything about how I thought about food — not as calories to count, but as information my body was responding to in real time.

### Why Glucose Matters for Weight Loss

Glucose isn't just about diabetes—it's the master key to understanding how your body stores and burns fat. Here's why:

**Insulin and Fat Storage**: When you eat, particularly foods high in carbohydrates, your blood glucose rises. In response, your pancreas releases insulin, a hormone that tells your cells to absorb glucose from the bloodstream. Insulin is also a powerful signal for fat storage. When insulin levels are high, your body is in "storage mode," making it nearly impossible to burn fat. When insulin levels are low, you can access stored fat for energy.

**The Glucose Roller Coaster**: Large spikes in blood glucose trigger large releases of insulin. What goes up must come down—and often these spikes are followed by crashes that leave you feeling hungry, tired, and craving more carbohydrates.

This creates a vicious cycle of eating, spiking, crashing, and eating again.

**Individual Variability**: Perhaps most importantly, people respond very differently to the same foods. A study from the Weizmann Institute found that glucose responses to identical meals varied dramatically between individuals—some people spiked from bananas but not cookies, while others showed the opposite pattern. A CGM reveals YOUR unique responses, not generic dietary advice.

**The Science Behind Glucose Variability**

Research has identified several factors that influence your glucose response to food:

- **Gut microbiome composition**: The trillions of bacteria in your digestive system affect how you metabolize different foods
- **Sleep quality**: Poor sleep increases insulin resistance and glucose variability
- **Stress levels**: Cortisol raises blood glucose even without eating
- **Exercise timing and intensity**: Movement affects how your muscles absorb glucose

- **Meal composition**: The combination of protein, fat, and fiber with carbohydrates
- **Meal timing**: The same food can produce different responses at different times of day
- **Genetics**: Your DNA plays a role in glucose metabolism

A CGM allows you to see all these factors in action in your own body.

# Chapter 3: Your First Two Weeks with a CGM

My first week with the CGM was humbling. I didn't change a single thing about how I ate — I just watched. And what I saw surprised me. Breakfast foods I'd considered healthy sent my glucose to 160. A walk after dinner flattened a spike that would have taken three hours to come down on its own. The first two weeks aren't about discipline — they're about discovery. Let the data do the talking before you change a thing.

## Week One: Establish Your Baseline

During your first week, don't change anything about your diet or lifestyle. This is your baseline period. The goal is to understand how your body currently responds to your normal eating patterns.

Each day in week one, log everything you eat including portions and timing, note how you feel one to two hours after each meal, check your morning fasting glucose, and take screenshots of anything that surprises you. You're not judging yet — you're just collecting evidence.

As the week unfolds, you're looking for a handful of key patterns: which foods produce the biggest spikes, which meals leave you feeling stable and satisfied versus foggy and hungry an hour later, when during the day your body handles carbohydrates most gracefully, and how your morning fasting glucose shifts depending on what you ate and how you slept the night before. These patterns are the raw material for everything you'll do in week two.

**Week Two: Begin Experiments**

Now start making strategic changes based on what you learned in week one.

Food pairing is where most people have their first genuine surprise. Take the food that spiked you worst in week one and eat it again — but this time, pair it with protein, fat, or fiber. Watch what happens to the curve. For most people, the spike shrinks dramatically. That's not willpower; that's biochemistry. The presence of fat and protein physically slows how fast glucose enters your blood. Timing experiments are often the most eye-opening. Try eating the same meal at different points in the day — many people are genuinely shocked to find that a lunch that barely moves their glucose causes a significant spike when eaten at 8 PM. Your insulin sensitivity is not constant; it follows a daily rhythm, and the CGM makes that rhythm visible in a way no food journal ever could.

Movement experiments are perhaps the most immediately motivating. Take a ten-minute walk after a meal that normally spikes you and watch the curve flatten in real time. Many people describe this as the moment the CGM goes from being an interesting gadget to feeling like a genuine superpower — you're watching your own biology respond to a decision you just made.

Finally, try eating the same meal in a different order. Vegetables and protein first, carbohydrates last. Compare the CGM trace to eating everything together or starting with the carbs. The research on this is consistent, and your own data will almost certainly confirm it: sequence alone can reduce a spike by thirty to forty percent without changing a single ingredient.

Keep detailed notes on all experiments so you can identify winning strategies.

## Chapter 4: Reading Your CGM Data

In my first few days with the CGM, I stared at the numbers like they were written in a foreign language. 94 mg/dL. Then 147. Then 83. What did any of it mean? It took me about a week to stop seeing isolated numbers and start seeing a story — a pattern that told me exactly how my body was handling what I ate, how I slept, and how stressed I was. This chapter teaches you to read that story fluently, so the data becomes insight rather than noise.

### Understanding the Numbers

For someone without diabetes, here are the glucose ranges you'll typically see:

- **Normal fasting glucose**: 70-100 mg/dL (3.9-5.6 mmol/L)
- **Target range throughout the day**: 70-120 mg/dL (3.9-6.7 mmol/L)
- **Acceptable post-meal peak**: Less than 140 mg/dL (7.8 mmol/L)
- **Optimal post-meal peak for metabolic health**: Less than 110 mg/dL (6.1 mmol/L)

For weight loss, you want to minimize both the height of glucose spikes and the total time spent above your baseline.

*Hypoglycemia awareness: Although non-diabetic individuals rarely experience dangerously low blood sugar, CGM use can occasionally reveal glucose dipping below 70 mg/dL. Symptoms of low blood sugar include shakiness, sweating, dizziness, confusion, heart palpitations, or sudden hunger. If you experience these symptoms, consume 15 grams of fast-acting carbohydrates (e.g., 4 oz juice or glucose tablets) and recheck your glucose in 15 minutes. If symptoms are severe or do not improve, seek immediate medical attention. If you are on any medications, including those not for diabetes, consult your physician, as some medications can affect glucose levels.*

> A note on targets: In the Quick Start Guide you will see an aspirational post-meal target of <120 mg/dL — that is the 'excellent' zone. The practical working goal for most people starting out is <130 mg/dL, which represents meaningful metabolic improvement without perfectionism. As your insulin sensitivity improves over weeks, <120 mg/dL becomes increasingly achievable as your new natural baseline. Start with <130 mg/dL; let <120 mg/dL become your goal over time.

**Understanding Post-Meal Glucose Spikes: What's Normal vs. What's Optimal**

**Important: Post-meal glucose spikes are completely normal.** When you eat, especially foods containing carbohydrates, your glucose will rise. This is your body's natural response to food, and it happens to everyone, even people with perfect metabolic health.

The key questions are: 1. **How high does it spike?** (Peak height)

2. **How quickly does it return to baseline?** (Recovery time)

Every post-meal response moves through four phases. In the first fifteen minutes, digestion begins and glucose starts entering your bloodstream. Over the next thirty to sixty minutes, it climbs to its peak as insulin is released to move glucose into your cells — this is when you'll see the highest reading on your CGM. Then comes the recovery: over the following sixty to ninety minutes, glucose descends back toward where it started as insulin clears it from the blood. Finally, ninety to a hundred and eighty minutes after eating, you return to baseline — the meal processed, insulin falling, your body ready for what comes next.

2. **How quickly does it return to baseline?** (Recovery time)

**What Happens During a Normal Post-Meal Response:**

**Eating Phase (0-15 minutes after eating)**:

- You finish your meal

- Digestion begins

- Glucose starts entering the bloodstream

**Peak Phase (30-60 minutes after eating)**:

- This is when you'll see your CGM reading at its maximum
- Insulin is released to move glucose into cells
- This is when you'll see your CGM reading at its maximum

**Recovery Phase (60-120 minutes after eating)**:

- Glucose begins declining back toward baseline
- Insulin is working to clear glucose from the blood
- Your body is processing the meal

**Return to Baseline (90-180 minutes after eating)**:

- Glucose returns to your pre-meal level

**The Critical Metrics: Peak Height and Recovery Time**

**Peak Height: How High Is Too High?**

**Metabolically Healthy Response:**

- **Excellent**: Peak stays under 110 mg/dL (rise of less than 20 mg/dL from baseline)

- **Good**: Peak stays under 120 mg/dL (rise of 20-30 mg/dL from baseline) - **Acceptable**: Peak stays under 140 mg/dL (rise of 30-50 mg/dL from baseline)

- **Concerning**: Peak exceeds 140 mg/dL (rise of more than 50 mg/dL from baseline)

- **Problematic**: Peak exceeds 160 mg/dL (rise of more than 70 mg/dL from baseline)

**Example**: - Your fasting glucose: 85 mg/dL - After breakfast, glucose peaks at 115 mg/dL

- **Rise**: 30 mg/dL (85 → 115)

- **Assessment**: Good response, minimal insulin spike

**Recovery Time: How Fast Should It Come Down?**

This is equally important as peak height. Even if you spike to 140 mg/dL, if you return to baseline quickly, the total insulin exposure is lower.

The recovery tiers work like this. An excellent recovery means your glucose returns to within 10 mg/dL of your pre-meal baseline within sixty to ninety minutes — a sign of strong insulin sensitivity. A good recovery takes ninety to a hundred and twenty minutes. Acceptable sits in the two-to-three-hour range, suggesting room to improve. If you're still elevated after three hours, or if glucose from one meal hasn't cleared before the next one begins, that points toward insulin resistance — which is exactly what this program is designed to reverse.

**Metabolically Healthy Recovery Times:**

**Excellent Recovery:**

- Returns to within 10 mg/dL of baseline in **60-90 minutes**
- Example: 85 → 120 → 90 mg/dL within 90 minutes
- This indicates excellent insulin sensitivity

**Good Recovery:**

- Returns to within 10 mg/dL of baseline in **90-120 minutes** (1.5-2 hours)
- Example: 85 → 130 → 95 mg/dL within 2 hours
- This indicates good insulin sensitivity

**Acceptable Recovery:**

- Returns to within 10 mg/dL of baseline in **120-180 minutes** (2-3 hours)
- Example: 85 → 140 → 95 mg/dL within 3 hours
- This indicates moderate insulin sensitivity, room for improvement

**Concerning Recovery:** - Takes **more than 180 minutes** (3+ hours) to return to baseline
- Example: 85 → 145 → still at 110 mg/dL after 3 hours

- Doesn't return to baseline before the next meal

**Problematic Recovery:**

- Doesn't return to baseline before the next meal

- Example: 85 → 150 → still at 120 mg/dL when you eat again

**Visual Example: Two Different Responses to the Same Meal**

**Person A (Excellent Metabolic Health):**

- Baseline: 85 mg/dL - 30 min post-meal: 105 mg/dL (peak)

- 60 min post-meal: 95 mg/dL

- 90 min post-meal: 87 mg/dL (back to baseline)

- **Assessment**: Peak rise of only 20 mg/dL, returned to baseline in 90 minutes

- **Insulin exposure**: Minimal

- **Fat burning**: Resumed quickly

- **Fat burning**: Resumed quickly

**Person B (Insulin Resistance):**

- Baseline: 95 mg/dL - 45 min post-meal: 165 mg/dL (peak)
- 90 min post-meal: 145 mg/dL - 120 min post-meal: 125 mg/dL
- 180 min post-meal: 105 mg/dL (still above baseline)
- **Assessment**: Peak rise of 70 mg/dL, hasn't returned to baseline after 3 hours
- **Insulin exposure**: Very high and prolonged
- **Fat burning**: Blocked for 3+ hours

**Same meal. Dramatically different metabolic responses.**

**What Your CGM Should Show for Optimal Weight Loss**

**The Ideal Post-Meal Pattern:**

**Within 30-60 minutes**:

- Glucose peaks at less than 30 mg/dL above your baseline
- Ideally less than 20 mg/dL rise

**Within 90-120 minutes**:

- Glucose returns to within 10 mg/dL of your pre-meal baseline
- You feel satisfied, not hungry or sluggish

**Before your next meal**:

- Glucose is back at baseline or lower

- You have stable energy - Minimal to no cravings

**Example of an Ideal Day:**

**Breakfast (7 AM)**: - Pre-meal: 85 mg/dL - Peak (8 AM): 105 mg/dL

- Return to baseline (9 AM): 87 mg/dL

**Lunch (12 PM)**: - Pre-meal: 85 mg/dL - Peak (1 PM): 110 mg/dL

- Return to baseline (2 PM): 88 mg/dL

**Dinner (6 PM)**: - Pre-meal: 85 mg/dL - Peak (7 PM): 115 mg/dL

- Return to baseline (8 PM): 87 mg/dL

**Bedtime (10 PM)**: 85 mg/dL **Fasting next morning (7 AM)**: 83 mg/dL

**This pattern indicates**: Excellent glucose control, minimal insulin spikes, maximum fat-burning time, optimal metabolic health.

**Why Both Metrics Matter: The Area Under the Curve**

It's not just about the peak—it's about the **total glucose exposure over time**.

**Scenario 1**: High peak (160 mg/dL) but quick recovery (90 minutes back to baseline)

**Scenario 2**: Moderate peak (130 mg/dL) but slow recovery (4 hours to return)

**Scenario 2 is worse** because even though the peak is lower, the prolonged elevation means more total insulin secretion and longer fat-storage mode.
**Best case**: Low peak + fast recovery = minimal insulin, maximum fat burning

**Worst case**: High peak + slow recovery = maximum insulin, prolonged fat storage

**The Recovery Time Goal for Weight Loss**

**Your Target**: Return to within 10 mg/dL of your pre-meal baseline within **2 hours** (120 minutes) of finishing your meal.

The two-hour target exists for practical reasons. It keeps insulin exposure time-limited, which means your body can return to fat-burning mode before your next meal. It prevents glucose from one meal stacking on top of the next, which is one of the most common reasons people's energy crashes in the afternoon. And consistently hitting this target is one of the clearest signals that your insulin sensitivity is improving. To get there: balance your meals, sequence vegetables and protein before carbs, take a post-meal walk, and keep portions honest.

**Your Target**: Return to within 10 mg/dL of your pre-meal baseline within **2 hours** (120 minutes) of finishing your meal.

**Why 2 hours?**

- Keeps insulin exposure time-limited
- Allows fat burning to resume before your next meal
- Prevents compounding glucose elevation throughout the day
- Indicates healthy insulin sensitivity

**How to Achieve This:**

- Balanced meals (see Principle 2)
- Food sequencing (see Principle 3)

**What to Do If You're Not Meeting This Target:**

- Appropriate portion sizes (see Non-Negotiable #2)

**What to Do If You're Not Meeting This Target:**

1. Check your meal composition—likely too many carbs, not enough protein/fat
2. Reduce carbohydrate portions
3. Take a post-meal walk

**The "New Normal" You're Creating**

The improvements come in stages, and they're worth knowing in advance so you recognize progress when it's happening. In weeks one and two, you're mostly gathering information — peaks in the range of forty to sixty points above baseline are common, and recovery may take two to four hours. Don't be discouraged; this is your starting line, not a verdict. By weeks three through six, the peaks begin to soften, and recovery tightens toward ninety to a hundred and fifty minutes. By weeks seven through twelve, most people find their peaks reliably under thirty points above baseline with recovery in ninety minutes or less. After month four, glucose control starts to feel almost automatic — not because the biology changed, but because the behaviors became second nature.

**Week 1-2**:

**Week 1-2**:

- Becoming aware of your current patterns
- Peaks might be 40-60 mg/dL above baseline
- Recovery taking 2-4 hours

**Week 3-6**:

- Peaks reducing to 30-40 mg/dL above baseline
- Recovery improving to 90-150 minutes
- More stable energy throughout the day

**Week 7-12**:

- Peaks consistently under 30 mg/dL above baseline
- Recovery within 90-120 minutes

- Minimal cravings, stable hunger

**Month 4+**:

- Peaks often under 20 mg/dL above baseline

**Remember**: You're not trying to prevent glucose from rising after meals—that's impossible and unnecessary. You're optimizing how high it rises and how quickly it returns to baseline. That's where the magic of weight loss and metabolic health happens.

- Effortless glucose control, your new metabolic baseline

**Visual Comparison: A Day in My Glucose Life, yes that's my data**

A Typical Day WITHOUT CGM-Based Principles

November 27, 2025 · Continuous Glucose Monitor Trace of Author

---

A Typical Day WITHOUT CGM-Based Principles

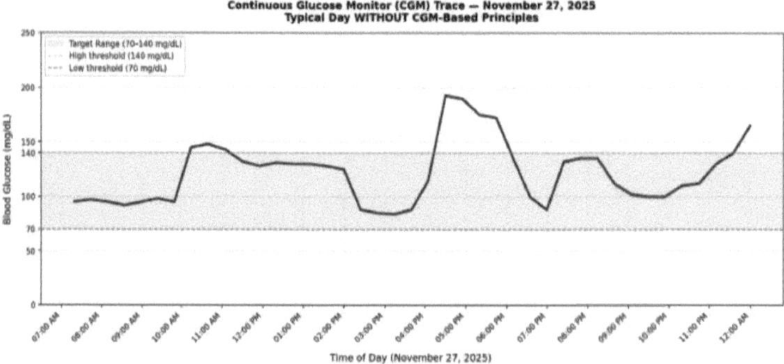


November 27, 2025 · Continuous Glucose Monitor Trace of Author

*Figure 1: CGM trace showing glucose instability throughout the day. Green band = target range (70–140 mg/dL).*

## Overview

This continuous glucose monitor (CGM) trace reveals a metabolically stressed day characterized by poor glucose regulation, significant post-meal excursions, and compounding instability across the full 24-hour window. The patterns observed are consistent with a day of unmanaged dietary choices that do not align with CGM-based principles for metabolic health.

### Key Findings

**1. High Fasting Glucose** (~90 mg/dL, ~7:00 AM)

The day begins already slightly elevated, suggesting poor previous-day dietary habits or evening hyperglycemia that prevented full overnight normalization. An ideal fasting glucose sits closer to 70–85 mg/dL. Waking above 90 mg/dL signals the body has not had adequate overnight recovery.

**2. First Post-Meal Spike** (~165 mg/dL, late morning)

The first major excursion climbs rapidly to approximately 165 mg/dL, indicating an unbalanced breakfast — likely high in refined carbohydrates with insufficient fiber, fat, or protein to blunt glucose absorption. This spike is sharp and fast, a hallmark of glycemic overload that stresses the pancreas and drives inflammation.

**3. Peak Hyperglycemia** (~190–194 mg/dL, ~4:30 PM)

The most alarming feature of the day. Glucose surges to nearly 194 mg/dL — well above the 140 mg/dL threshold considered the upper limit of a healthy post-meal response. This level is associated with oxidative stress, endothelial damage over time, and significant fatigue in the hours that follow.

**4. Slow Recovery** — 3+ Hours Above 140 mg/dL

Rather than returning to baseline within 90–120 minutes (a sign of good insulin sensitivity), glucose remains elevated for over three hours across the midday and afternoon window. This prolonged elevation suggests reduced insulin sensitivity, meaning cells are not efficiently clearing glucose from the bloodstream.

**5. Reactive Glucose Crash** (~83–85 mg/dL, ~3:00 PM)

Following the large midday spike, glucose drops sharply to the low-to-mid 80s — a reactive hypoglycemic dip driven by the exaggerated insulin response to the earlier surge. While not clinically hypoglycemic, this rapid fall typically causes intense cravings, brain fog, irritability, and fatigue, driving the urge to snack on high-carb foods and restart the cycle.

**6. Afternoon Re-Elevation** (~125–130 mg/dL, mid-afternoon)

Glucose climbs again into the mid-120s to 130 mg/dL range for an extended plateau — likely from a meal or snack consumed during the post-crash craving window. This keeps the body in a near-continuous state of mild hyperglycemia throughout the afternoon, with no meaningful return to baseline.

**7. Evening Spike** (~145–148 mg/dL, ~10:00–10:30 PM)

A late elevation reaching 145–148 mg/dL indicates an evening meal that was too carbohydrate-dense or consumed too late in the day. Evening hyperglycemia is particularly damaging because glucose clearance is naturally slower at night, and elevated glucose disrupts sleep architecture, growth hormone release, and overnight cellular repair.

**8. Worsening Next-Day Fasting Glucose** (~95–98 mg/dL)

By the final hours of the trace in the early morning, fasting glucose has risen to 95–98 mg/dL — measurably worse than the starting point of ~90 mg/dL. This is the compounding debt effect: poor glucose management today directly degrades the metabolic baseline tomorrow, creating a worsening cycle if repeated day after day.

# A Typical Day WITH CGM-Based Principles

December 9, 2025 · Continuous Glucose Monitor Trace of Author

---

A Typical Day WITH CGM-Based Principles

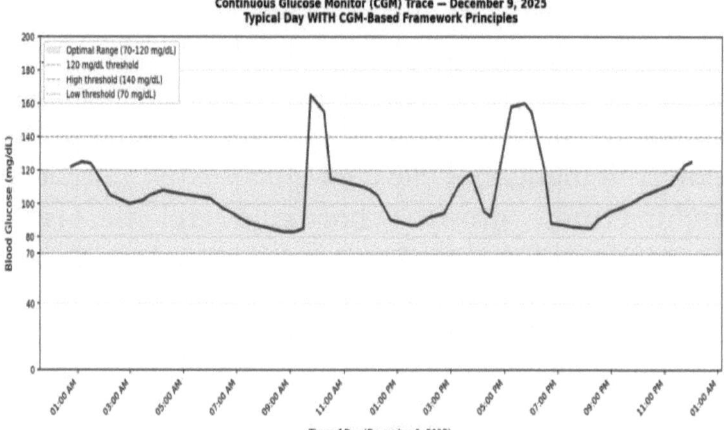


December 9, 2025 · Continuous Glucose Monitor Trace of Author

*Figure 2: CGM trace showing stable glucose regulation throughout the day. Green band = optimal range (70–120 mg/dL). This is the SAME person as Figure 1, following all framework principles.*

## Overview

This continuous glucose monitor (CGM) trace from December 9, 2025, represents the same individual shown in Figure 1 — but on a day where all CGM-based framework principles were applied. The contrast is striking. Where the previous day showed wild excursions reaching 194 mg/dL and 6+ hours above 140 mg/dL, this trace demonstrates what optimized metabolic function looks like: controlled post-meal responses, rapid recovery, stable energy, and an improving baseline from one morning to the next.

### Key Findings

**1. Optimal Fasting Glucose** (82 mg/dL, Early Morning)

The day opens with a fasting glucose of approximately 82 mg/dL — comfortably within the optimal 70–85 mg/dL range. This is a direct result of disciplined choices the previous day: balanced evening meals consumed early enough for overnight clearance, consistent sleep timing, and avoiding late-night eating. Waking at 82 mg/dL means the metabolic system is well-rested and primed for clean glucose handling throughout the day.

**2. Small, Controlled Post-Meal Spikes** (115–160 mg/dL)

Post-meal glucose peaks are visible but markedly restrained, reaching 115–160 mg/dL versus the 165–194 mg/dL seen on the unmanaged day. This reflects meals structured around the framework: fiber and protein consumed before carbohydrates, portion-appropriate carbohydrate loads, and adequate fat to slow gastric emptying. The shape of each spike is also gentler — a gradual rise rather than a sharp vertical climb — indicating the meal composition is working as intended.

**3. Fast Recovery** — 90 Minutes to Baseline

Following each post-meal peak, glucose returns to baseline within approximately 90 minutes. This is the hallmark signature of excellent insulin sensitivity. The pancreas is releasing an appropriate amount of insulin, cells are responding efficiently, and glucose is being cleared from circulation at a healthy rate. Compare this to the 3+ hour recovery times seen in Figure 1 — the difference reflects a fundamentally more responsive metabolic state.

**4. Stable Energy** — No Crashes or Cravings

Throughout the day, glucose never dips below approximately 83 mg/dL. There are no reactive hypoglycemic crashes following meal spikes — the pattern that drove intense cravings and rebound snacking in the unmanaged day. This stability is felt experientially as consistent mental clarity, sustained physical energy, and an absence of the mid-afternoon slump that is commonly misattributed to a need for caffeine or sugar.

**5. Minimal Time Above 120 mg/dL** (Under 2 Hours Total)

Total time above 120 mg/dL across the entire day is estimated at under two hours — the brief windows immediately following meals. In contrast, the unmanaged day showed approximately six hours above 140 mg/dL. Reducing time in elevated glucose states is directly associated with lower oxidative stress, reduced glycation of proteins, better vascular health, and improved cognitive function over the long term.

**6. Return to Baseline Before Sleep**

Glucose settles back into the 100–110 mg/dL range in the evening and continues declining toward the overnight low. This clean return to baseline before sleep means the body can devote overnight metabolic resources to cellular repair, growth hormone secretion, and immune function — all of which are compromised when blood glucose remains elevated into the sleep window. This pattern directly enables the improved fasting glucose seen the following morning.

## 7. Improving Next-Day Fasting Glucose (80 mg/dL)

By the final readings of the trace, the trajectory is clearly downward — projecting a next-morning fasting glucose of approximately 80 mg/dL, two points lower than this morning's 82 mg/dL. This illustrates the positive compounding effect that mirrors the negative compounding seen in Figure 1. Good choices today make tomorrow's starting conditions slightly better, and that small improvement compounds over days, weeks, and months into meaningfully different metabolic health outcomes.

By the final readings of the trace, the trajectory is clearly downward — projecting a next-morning fasting glucose of approximately 80 mg/dL, two points lower than this morning's 82 mg/dL. This illustrates the positive compounding effect that mirrors the negative compounding seen in Figure. Good choices today make tomorrow's starting conditions slightly better, and that small improvement compounds over days, weeks, and months into meaningfully different metabolic health outcomes.

## Framework Principles Applied on This Day

The glucose pattern shown in Figure 2 is consistent with the following evidence-based CGM framework principles being in effect throughout the day:

- Meal sequencing: fiber and protein consumed before carbohydrates to blunt absorption rate
- Balanced macronutrient composition: sufficient dietary fat and protein to slow gastric emptying
- Post-meal movement: light walking or activity within 30 minutes of eating to accelerate glucose uptake
- Early dinner timing: final meal consumed at least 3 hours before sleep to allow full overnight clearance
- Consistent sleep schedule: supporting circadian-aligned glucose metabolism and cortisol regulation
- Stress management: avoiding cortisol-driven fasting glucose spikes through mindfulness or structured recovery practices

**Consistent sleep schedule: supporting circadian-aligned glucose metabolism and cortisol regulation**

**The Bottom Line**: This is the same person, the same genetics, the same metabolism—just different behaviors. The framework doesn't change who you are; it changes how you support your body. The results speak for themselves.

**Key Metrics to Track**

**Average Glucose**: Your mean glucose level over a day or week. For weight loss, aim for an average between 90-100 mg/dL.

**Glucose Variability**: The standard deviation or coefficient of variation in your glucose readings. Lower variability generally indicates better metabolic health. Aim to keep your standard deviation under 15-20 mg/dL.

**Time in Range**: The percentage of time your glucose stays within your target range (typically 70-120 mg/dL). Aim for 90% or higher.

**Peak Heights**: How high your glucose spikes after meals. For weight loss, try to keep peaks under 30 mg/dL above baseline (ideally under 20 mg/dL).

**Area Under the Curve (AUC)**: The total glucose exposure over time, which correlates with insulin secretion. Smaller AUC means less insulin and more fat burning.

**Patterns to Look For**

**Dawn Phenomenon**: Many people see glucose rise in the early morning hours (4-8 AM) even without eating, due to cortisol and other hormones. This is normal but can be reduced with better sleep, stress management, and evening exercise.

**Reactive Hypoglycemia**: When glucose spikes high and then crashes below baseline, causing intense hunger and cravings. This pattern is a major obstacle to weight loss.

**Prolonged Elevation**: Glucose that stays elevated for hours after a meal suggests insulin resistance and poor metabolic health.

**Flat and Stable**: The ideal pattern—minimal spikes, quick returns to baseline, and stable glucose throughout the day.

## Chapter 5: The 10 Principles of CGM-Based Weight Loss

If I had to distill everything I learned from three months of CGM data into a single sentence, it would be this: your body is not random. Every spike, every flat line, every crash has a cause — and once you know the causes, you can change the outcomes. The ten principles in this chapter are the ones that showed up, consistently, in my data and in the research. They're not rules to follow perfectly; they're levers to pull, one at a time, until your glucose tells you it's working.

**Principle 1: Minimize Glucose Spikes**

The single most important principle for weight loss is keeping glucose stable. Every spike trigger insulin release, and insulin blocks fat burning while promoting fat storage.

In practice, aim to keep post-meal increases under 30 mg/dL above your baseline. If a food consistently pushes you over that threshold, that's not a moral failing — it's a data point. Try reducing the portion, adding fat or protein alongside it, eating it earlier in the day, or pairing it with a short walk. The CGM tells you whether the adjustment worked. You iterate until it does.

**Principle 2: Optimize Meal Composition**

The combination of macronutrients matters enormously. Carbohydrates alone spike glucose rapidly, but when combined with protein, fat, and fiber, the response is blunted.

**The Glucose-Stable Plate**: - 40-50% non-starchy vegetables (fiber) - 25-30% protein - 15-

20% healthy fats - 5-15% complex carbohydrates (if any)

**Practical Application**: Test different ratios and see what keeps you stable. Some people do better with very low carbs; others can handle moderate amounts when properly paired.

**Principle 3: Sequence Your Foods**

The order in which you eat foods during a meal significantly affects your glucose response. Studies in people with type 2 diabetes show that eating vegetables and protein before carbohydrates can meaningfully reduce the post-meal glucose spike — with reductions of around 40% reported in some controlled trials. Results vary between individuals, and the effect in non-diabetic adults is likely smaller, but your CGM will show you your own response clearly. [Imai et al., 2014, Diabetes Care; Shukla et al., 2017, Diabetes Care, 38(7), e98–e99. [PubMed: 25931478]]

The optimal sequence is vegetables first, then protein and fat, then carbohydrates last. It sounds almost too simple to matter, but the research is consistent and your CGM will confirm it in your own body. Fiber from the vegetables physically coats the gut, slowing glucose absorption for everything that follows. When carbohydrates arrive last, they enter a system already primed to handle them gently.

**Practical Application**: Use your CGM to test this. Eat a typical meal in your normal way, then a few days later eat the exact same meal but, in the vegetable, →protein→carb sequence. Compare the glucose curves.

**Principle 4: Time Your Eating Window**

When you eat matters almost as much as what you eat. Most people show higher insulin sensitivity in the morning and become more insulin resistant as the day progresses.

Consider confining your eating to an eight-to-twelve-hour window — something like 8 AM to 6 PM. This creates a meaningful fasting period each night where insulin stays low and fat burning can proceed uninterrupted. Front-load your calories toward earlier in the day when insulin sensitivity is at its highest. Many people are surprised to find that a carbohydrate serving they handle comfortably at noon causes a significant spike at 8 PM — not because the food changed, but because their body's capacity to process it diminished as the day went on.

**Time-Restricted Eating**: Consider confining you're eating to an 8–12-hour window, such as 8

AM to 6 PM. This provides a daily fasting period that allows insulin levels to drop and fat burning to occur.

**Front-Load Your Calories**: Your CGM will likely show that you handle carbohydrates better earlier in the day. Consider making breakfast or lunch your largest meal.

**Principle 5: Move After Meals**

Physical activity, especially after eating, helps your muscles absorb glucose without requiring as much insulin. Even gentle movement makes a dramatic difference.

**The Post-Meal Walk: Your Most Powerful Tool**

If you implement only one strategy from this entire book, make it this one: **take a brisk 30-minute walk after EVERY major meal—breakfast, lunch, and dinner**. Research consistently shows that post-meal walking significantly reduces the height and duration of glucose spikes compared to remaining sedentary — with studies reporting meaningful reductions in post-meal glucose and insulin levels. Your own CGM will show you the effect in real time. [Colberg et al., 2009, Diabetes Care; Reynolds et al., 2016, Diabetologia]

**The Complete Daily Protocol**: - 30 minutes after breakfast - 30 minutes after lunch - 30 minutes after dinner - **Total: 90 minutes of walking per day**

This may sound like a lot but remember you're breaking it into three manageable 30-minute sessions that happen naturally after you eat. These aren't extra activities crammed into your day—they're integrated into the rhythm of your meals.

**Why 30 Minutes After Each Meal?**

Research shows that 30 minutes of moderate activity post-meal provides optimal glucose control benefits. The first 10 minutes help but continuing to 30 minutes maximizes muscle glucose uptake and keeps insulin levels lower for hours afterward.

Walking after all three major meals creates a compound effect: - **Breakfast walk**: Sets stable glucose for the morning, improves focus and energy - **Lunch walk**: Prevents afternoon energy crash and cravings - **Dinner walk**: Most critical—prevents overnight glucose elevation, improves sleep, enhances morning fasting glucose

**What "Brisk" Means**: - Purposeful, not strolling - You can talk but should feel slightly breathless - Heart rate elevated but comfortable -

About 3-4 mph (faster than window shopping, slower than racing)

**Practical Examples by Meal**:

**After Breakfast** (30 minutes | 7-8 AM): - Walk around your neighborhood before starting work (establish this as your morning routine) - If working from home, walk while taking a phone call or listening to news/podcast - Park farther from your office and walk the rest of the way - Use a treadmill desk or walking pad while checking emails - Walk your kids to school instead of driving - Walk to get your morning coffee instead of making it at home

**After Lunch** (30 minutes | 12-1 PM): - Take a walking meeting with colleagues (increasingly common and productive) - Walk to a nearby park and back during your lunch break - Walk to get your lunch instead of using delivery - Walk laps around your office building or parking lot - Use stairs for the entire 30 minutes (extremely effective) - Walk to run a quick errand during lunch hour

**After Dinner** (30 minutes | 6-8 PM): - Walk with your spouse or partner—make it daily conversation time and connection - Walk your dog (or offer to walk a neighbor's dog) - Listen to a podcast, audiobook, or music while walking solo - Walk to a nearby destination (coffee shop, bookstore, friend's house) - Evening family walk as a wind-down ritual before bedtime routine - Walk around your neighborhood to see neighbors and build community

**The CGM Evidence You'll See**:

Your glucose curve will show this in real-time after each meal:

**Without post-meal walk**: - Glucose peaks at 160 mg/dL at 45 minutes post-meal - Takes 3 hours to return to baseline - Area under the curve: high insulin exposure - **Three meals without walks = 9+ hours of elevated glucose daily** **With 30-minute post-meal walk after each meal**: - Glucose peaks at 120 mg/dL at 30 minutes post-meal - Returns to baseline within 90 minutes - Area under the curve: substantially lower insulin exposure - **Three walks = significantly reduced daily insulin exposure and enhanced fat burning**

This is the power of movement—and you can see it happening in your body in real-time after every single meal.

**Building the Habit**: How to Actually Do This

**Week 1-2**: Start with ONE meal - Choose dinner (most important for overnight metabolism) - Make it non-negotiable: eat dinner, then immediately walk - Build the automatic connection: dinner = walk

**Week 3-4**: Add the SECOND meal - Add lunch walks to your routine - Now: lunch = walk, dinner = walk - Two meals down, glucose control improving significantly

**Week 5-6**: Add the THIRD meal - Add breakfast walks - All three meals now trigger automatic walking - Full protocol in place: breakfast = walk, lunch = walk, dinner = walk

**Week 7+**: This is your new lifestyle - Walking after meals feels as automatic as brushing your teeth - You feel restless if you DON'T walk after eating - Your CGM has retrained your brain to crave post-meal movement

**Best Practices**: - Start walking within 15-30 minutes of finishing your meal (ideally within 15 minutes) - Consistency matters more than intensity—daily walks at moderate pace beat occasional intense exercise - Don't skip even if the meal was small or "healthy"—the habit matters as much as the glucose benefit - Make it enjoyable: good shoes, pleasant route, company or entertainment

**When You Can't Walk for 30 Minutes After Every Meal**:

Life happens. Here are effective strategies:

**Minimum Viable Protocol**: - 10 minutes after each meal is still powerful (30 min/day total) - Even 5 minutes after each meal provides benefits (15 min/day total) - Any walking is better than no walking

**Priority Ranking** (if you must choose): 1. **Dinner** (most important—affects overnight glucose and morning readings) 2. **Lunch** (prevents afternoon crashes and evening overeating) 3. **Breakfast** (sets the day's metabolic tone)

**Movement Snacks** (if you can't take 30 continuous minutes): - 10 minutes right after eating - 10 minutes mid-morning/afternoon/evening - 10 minutes before your next meal - Total: 30 minutes per meal period, just not continuous (still quite effective!)

**Alternative Movements** (if walking isn't possible): - Bodyweight squats: 3 sets of 15-20 reps - Stair climbing: 10-15 minutes - Dancing: Put on music and move vigorously - Household chores: Vacuuming, gardening, cleaning (if vigorous) - Playing actively with kids or pets - Cycling (stationary or outdoor) - Swimming

**Advanced Strategy**: Strength Training Before Meals

Strength training before a meal can increase insulin sensitivity for hours afterward, allowing you to handle more carbohydrates without the same glucose spike.

**Example Protocol**: - 20-30 minutes of strength training in the late afternoon (4-5 PM) - Dinner 30-60 minutes after training (5:30-6:30 PM) - Walk after dinner (7-7:30 PM) - Your CGM will show significantly blunted glucose response to the same meal

This is especially useful for special occasions when you know you'll be eating more carbohydrates than usual.

**The 90-Minute Question: "I Don't Have Time"**

Let's address this directly: 90 minutes of walking spread across breakfast, lunch, and dinner is the single most powerful intervention for weight loss and metabolic health. More powerful than any supplement, any specific diet, any bio hack.

**Time-Finding Strategies**:

1. **It's already break time**: You're taking breaks after meals anyway. Walk instead of scrolling.
2. **Combine with existing activities**:

– Walk while on phone calls (work or personal)

– Walk to accomplish errands

– Walk as family time or dog time (things you'd do anyway)

3. **Replace sedentary time**:

   – 90 minutes of walking replaces 90 minutes of sitting

   – You're not adding 90 minutes to your day—you're changing what you do during those 90 minutes

4. **Consider the ROI**:

   – 90 minutes of walking = weight loss, better sleep, more energy, clearer thinking, lower stress

   – Would you "spend" 90 minutes to feel dramatically better and lose weight? Most people spend more time than that on social media daily.

**The Bottom Line**:

If you do nothing else from this entire book, walk for 30 minutes after breakfast, lunch, and dinner. Your CGM will show you within days that this works. Your body will show you within weeks with weight loss, better energy, and reduced cravings.

This is the foundation. Everything else optimizes it. But this alone can transform your metabolic health.

**Principle 6: Prioritize Sleep**

Poor sleep is one of the fastest ways to disrupt glucose control. Research consistently shows that even a single night of poor sleep meaningfully increases insulin resistance and raises fasting glucose. Controlled studies have found reductions in insulin sensitivity of around 25–30% following sleep restriction, though individual responses vary. [Spiegel et al., 1999, The Lancet; Donga et al., 2010, J Clin Endocrinol Metab]

**Sleep and Glucose**: Your CGM will show higher baseline glucose and more variability on days after poor sleep. You'll also experience more cravings and larger spikes from the same foods.

**The Non-Negotiable Target**: 7-9 hours of quality sleep per night, on a consistent schedule. This isn't optional—it's foundational to everything else in this book.

**The Sleep-Glucose Connection You'll See on Your CGM**:

**After Poor Sleep (5-6 hours)** (representative example — individual responses vary): - Fasting glucose: 95–105 mg/dL (normally 85–90 mg/dL) - Breakfast spike: up to 150 mg/dL (normally around 120 mg/dL) - Higher glucose variability all day - Prolonged elevation after meals - Increased cravings for high-carb foods

**After Good Sleep (7-9 hours)**: - Fasting glucose: 80-90 mg/dL - Breakfast spike: 110 mg/dL - Stable glucose throughout the day - Quick return to baseline after meals - Reduced hunger and cravings

The difference is dramatic and immediate—your CGM doesn't lie about the importance of sleep.

**Optimize Sleep for Metabolic Health**:

**1. Consistent Sleep Schedule** - Go to bed at the same time every night (even weekends) - Wake up at the same time every morning - Your body's circadian rhythm synchronizes insulin sensitivity with this schedule - Inconsistent sleep confuses your metabolism

**Example Schedule**: - Weekdays: Sleep 10 PM - 6 AM (8 hours) - Weekends: Sleep 10 PM - 6 AM (maintain consistency) - Avoid the temptation to "catch up" on weekends—consistency is more important than duration

**2. Stop Eating 3 Hours Before Bed** - Late-night eating elevates glucose during sleep - Your body should be fasting and repairing during sleep, not digesting - Evening glucose elevation impairs sleep quality

**Example**: - If you sleep at 10 PM, finish dinner by 7 PM - If you sleep at 11 PM, finish dinner by 8 PM - Light herbal tea or water is fine; food is not

**3. Create a Dark, Cool Sleep Environment** - Temperature: 65-68°F (18-20°C) is optimal - Complete darkness: Use blackout curtains or an eye mask - No light from devices, alarm clocks, or streetlights - blue light suppresses melatonin and disrupts circadian rhythm

**Example Bedroom Setup**: - Blackout curtains or shades - Cover or remove LED lights from electronics - Use a dim red nightlight if needed (doesn't disrupt melatonin) - Keep phone in another room or in airplane mode

**4. No Screens 1 Hour Before Bed** - Blue light from phones, tablets, TVs, and computers signals "daytime" to your brain - This suppresses melatonin and delays sleep onset - Even with blue light filters, the stimulation keeps your mind active

**Evening Screen-Free Activities**: - Read a physical book - Practice gentle stretching or yoga -

Journal or write - Have conversations with family - Listen to calming music or podcasts (audio only) - Meditate or practice deep breathing

**Example Evening Routine**: - 8:00 PM: Finish dinner - 8:30 PM: Clean up, prepare for next day - 9:00 PM: All screens off, dim lights in house - 9:00-9:30 PM: Evening stretching routine (10-15 minutes) - 9:30-10:00 PM: Read in bed with warm, dim lighting - 10:00 PM: Lights out, sleep

**5. No Caffeine After 2 PM** - Caffeine has a half-life of 5-6 hours - Coffee at 4 PM means half the caffeine is still in your system at 10 PM - Even if you "can" fall asleep with caffeine, it reduces deep sleep quality

**Caffeine Guidelines**: - Morning coffee: Fine (even beneficial for glucose control in some people) - Afternoon coffee (after 2 PM): Switch to decaf or herbal tea - Evening: No caffeine whatsoever - Test with your CGM: Some people show elevated morning glucose after late caffeine

**6. Get Morning Sunlight Exposure** - Natural light within 30 minutes of waking sets your circadian rhythm - This improves nighttime melatonin production 12-14 hours later - 10-15 minutes of outdoor light is sufficient (even on cloudy days)

**Morning Light Examples**: - Take your post-breakfast walk outside - Have coffee on your porch or balcony - Open curtains and sit by a window (less effective but better than nothing) - Walk your dog first thing in the morning

**7. Evening Wind-Down Routine** - Consistent pre-sleep routine signals your body it's time to rest - Include calming activities that lower cortisol - Make it enjoyable so you look forward to it

**Sample Wind-Down Routines**:

**Option 1 (60 minutes)**: - 9:00 PM: Dim all lights, change into sleepwear - 9:10 PM: Evening stretching routine (10 minutes) - 9:20 PM: Warm shower or bath - 9:35 PM: Skin care routine - 9:40 PM: Reading in bed - 10:00 PM: Sleep

**Option 2 (45 minutes)**: - 9:15 PM: Prepare for next day (lay out clothes, pack lunch) - 9:30 PM: Light stretching or yoga - 9:45 PM: Meditation or deep breathing (10 minutes) - 9:55 PM: Journaling or gratitude practice - 10:00 PM: Sleep

**Option 3 (30 minutes)**: - 9:30 PM: All screens off - 9:35 PM: Quick stretch routine (5 minutes) - 9:40 PM: Read in bed - 10:00 PM: Sleep

**8. Track Sleep and Glucose Correlation** - Use your CGM data alongside sleep tracking - Most sleep trackers or apps can log sleep duration and quality - Notice the direct relationship between sleep quality and next-day glucose

**What to Track**: - Sleep duration (hours) - Sleep quality (subjective rating 1-10) - Next-day fasting glucose - Next-day glucose variability - Next-day energy and cravings

**You'll likely discover**: - Every hour of sleep under 7 raises fasting glucose by 5-10 mg/dL - Poor sleep increases glucose spikes by 20-30 mg/dL - Weekend sleep inconsistency disrupts Monday-Tuesday glucose control

**When Sleep Is Difficult**:

If you struggle with sleep despite good practices:

**Common Issues and Solutions**: - **Can't fall asleep**: practice 4-7-8 breathing - **Wake up frequently**: Address late eating, reduce evening fluids, check room temperature - **Wake up tired**: May indicate sleep apnea—consult a doctor - **Racing thoughts**: Journal before bed to "download" worries, practice meditation - **Stress and anxiety**: Address through the self-compassion practices in Principle 7

**Medical Consultation**: If sleep problems persist despite optimization, consult a healthcare provider. Sleep disorders (apnea, restless leg syndrome, insomnia) significantly impair glucose control and require professional treatment.

**The Sleep-First Approach**:
Here's a powerful truth: if you had to choose between perfect eating and perfect sleep, choose sleep. Good sleep makes healthy eating easier. Poor sleep makes healthy eating nearly impossible.

When you're well-rested: - Cravings decrease - Willpower is stronger - Glucose stays stable - Fat burning increases - Exercise feels easier - Stress management is simpler

Sleep is the foundation. Protect it fiercely.

**Principle 7: Manage Stress**

Psychological stress triggers cortisol release, which raises blood glucose even without eating. Chronic stress promotes insulin resistance and weight gain.

**Stress-Glucose Connection**: Your CGM may show glucose spikes during stressful work meetings, difficult conversations, or anxiety-provoking situations. This is your body preparing for "fight or flight" by mobilizing energy.

**Stress Management Strategies**: - Practice daily meditation or deep breathing - Regular exercise (which also improves glucose control) -

Time in nature - Social connection - Adequate sleep (see Principle 6)

**Practical Application**: Note stressful events and check your CGM afterward. This awareness can be powerful motivation to develop better stress management practices.

*A Journey from Self-Doubt to Self-Love: A Stress Management Framework*

One of the most profound ways to manage stress is to transform your relationship with yourself. Chronic self-criticism and perfectionism are significant sources of cortisol elevation and glucose dysregulation. This framework offers a path to inner peace that directly supports your metabolic health.

**The Beginning: Recognizing Beauty in Flaws**

The journey begins with a transformative realization about your own reflection. Many people spend years fixating on perceived imperfections—whether physical, behavioral, or related to their weight loss journey. The act of seeing good qualities amidst flaws becomes the first step toward inner peace.

When you stop obsessing over the number on the scale or the glucose spike you had yesterday, you create space for self-acceptance. This doesn't mean giving up on your goals; it means accepting yourself as you are right now, rather than who you think you should be.

**Your CGM Practice**: When you see a glucose spike that frustrates you, pause. Instead of self-criticism ("I can't believe I ate that!"), practice observation ("My glucose spiked to 145 mg/dL after that meal. What can I learn from this?"). This shifts you from judgment to curiosity.

### Discovering Stillness

A shift occurs as calmness is found within. The exhausting cycle of constantly pushing, forcing, and rushing through life—including your weight loss efforts—comes to an end. Self-care becomes a priority rather than an afterthought.

Many people approach weight loss with frantic energy: strict meal plans, punishing exercise, constant monitoring, harsh self-talk when they "slip up." This approach elevates cortisol, disrupts glucose, and is ultimately unsustainable.

Instead, discover the power of stillness. Your weight loss journey doesn't require constant hustle. Sometimes the most productive thing you can do is rest, breathe, and simply be.

**Your CGM Practice**: Use your glucose data as a tool for gentle self-discovery, not a weapon for self-flagellation. When you notice elevated morning glucose after poor sleep, the response isn't "I'm failing," but "My body is asking for better rest." Honor that message.

**Befriending Yourself**

One of life's most challenging emotions is loneliness, and it's often heightened during weight loss when you feel different from others, restricted, or isolated in your health journey. A powerful truth emerges loneliness loses its sting when you become your own companion.

Learning to talk to yourself with kindness replaces harsh self-criticism. Self-love emerges not as narcissism, but as essential friendship with oneself. When you're your own friend, you encourage yourself during setbacks, celebrate small victories, and offer comfort during struggles.

**Your CGM Practice**: Notice your internal dialogue when reviewing your glucose data. Would you speak to a friend the way you speak to yourself? If not, consciously shift to a compassionate voice. "My glucose was high all day" becomes "I'm learning what my body needs and today gave me valuable information."

### Embracing the Unfinished

There's tenderness toward failures and incomplete efforts. Rather than shame when you don't follow the plan perfectly, these imperfect days receive compassion. The focus shifts from reaching destinations (goal weight, perfect glucose curves) to trusting the journey itself.

Weight loss is not linear. Glucose patterns vary daily. Some days you'll eat perfectly and still spike. Other days you'll eat imperfectly and feel fine. This is the human experience. Perfectionism is the enemy of progress.

**Your CGM Practice**: Keep a "learning log" instead of a "failure log." When something doesn't go as planned, write: "Today I learned that stress affects my glucose as much as food" or "I discovered that I could enjoy a small portion of dessert after a protein-rich meal without significant impact." Every data point is valuable, even the ones that don't match your expectations.

### Liberation from External Validation

The final theme celebrates breaking free from others' opinions. Many people spend years hating their bodies through the lens of external judgment—cultural beauty standards, family comments, social media comparisons, diet culture messaging.

Finding joy even when criticized for "flying too high" becomes important. When others comment on your food choices, your body, or your approach to health, their opinions reflect their own relationship with food and body—not your worth or your path.

**Your CGM Practice**: Your glucose data is yours alone. What works for someone else's metabolism may not work for yours. Trust your own data over generic advice or someone else's "miracle diet." You are the expert on your own body.

**A Crucial Balance: The Wisdom of Rest**

While this journey celebrates breaking free from rushing and forcing, it's equally important to remember that "flying too high" without rest can become its own form of self-harm. Doing too much—even in pursuit of health goals—can lead to burnout, disconnection from your body's needs, and ironically, the same kind of self-abandonment you worked to overcome.

Overexercising to "compensate" for a meal, obsessively checking your CGM every five minutes, restricting food to dangerous levels, or becoming so rigid about glucose control that you can't enjoy life—these are not self-love. They are new forms of the old self-punishment.

True self-love means honoring your limits, recognizing when ambition becomes self-destruction, and understanding that rest isn't laziness—it's wisdom. Your body needs recovery days. Your mind needs breaks from data. Your soul needs pleasure, connection, and foods eaten simply for joy sometimes.

Balance, not extremes in either direction, is where sustainable peace lives.

**Integrating This Practice with Your CGM Journey**

Each week, spend 10 minutes journaling on these questions:

1. **Self-Acceptance**: What did I appreciate about myself this week, regardless of my glucose patterns or weight?
2. **Stillness**: When did I choose rest over pushing myself too hard? How did my body respond?
3. **Self-Friendship**: How did I speak to myself during challenging moments? Can I speak kindlier?

4. **Embracing Imperfection**: What "imperfect" day taught me something valuable?
5. **Inner Validation**: Did I make any choices based on my own data and needs rather than external pressure?

This framework doesn't just reduce stress—it fundamentally changes your relationship with the weight loss process. When you approach your health from a place of self-compassion rather than self-criticism, cortisol decreases, glucose stabilizes, and paradoxically, the weight often comes off more easily because you're no longer fighting yourself.

Your CGM becomes a tool of self-discovery and self-love, not a judge and jury. And that shift changes everything.

**Principle 8: Stay Hydrated**

Dehydration concentrates your blood, making glucose readings appear higher. It also impairs your kidneys' ability to excrete excess glucose. Proper hydration supports metabolic health.

Drink water consistently throughout the day, aiming for pale yellow urine as your guide. Increase intake during exercise and in hot weather. Before you investigate a high fasting glucose reading, ask whether you were well-hydrated the day before —

many people discover a five-to-ten-point difference between dehydrated and properly hydrated readings, which can create false alarms if you don't account for it.

**Practical Application**: Test your fasting glucose when well-hydrated versus dehydrated. Many people see a 5-10 mg/dL difference.

**Principle 9: Choose the Right Carbohydrates**

Not all carbohydrates are created equal. Your CGM will reveal which ones you tolerate well, and which cause problematic spikes.

For most people, legumes — lentils, chickpeas, black beans — produce relatively modest glucose responses thanks to their fiber and protein content. Steel-cut or rolled oats tend to behave better than instant varieties. Sweet potatoes, quinoa, and most berries are generally well-tolerated in moderate portions. White bread, white rice, regular pasta, breakfast cereals, and anything made with refined flour tend to produce larger spikes more quickly. But "for most people" is not the same as "for you." Some individuals spike dramatically on oatmeal and handle white rice surprisingly well. Your CGM resolves this individual variation in a way that no food chart can.

**Lower-Spike Carbohydrates** (for most people): - Legumes (lentils, chickpeas, black beans) - Steel-cut or rolled oats (not instant) - Quinoa - Sweet potatoes - Most fruits (especially berries) - Whole grains in moderation

**Practical Application**: Test different carbohydrate sources in controlled portions and compare the responses. You may be surprised—some people spike from oatmeal but not rice, or vice versa. Build your diet around the carbs YOU tolerate best.

**Principle 10: Create Personalized Food Rules**

After several weeks of CGM data, you'll have clear insights into which foods support your weight loss goals, and which don't. Create simple, personal guidelines based on this data.

**Example Personal Rules**: - "I can have berries with breakfast without spiking" - "Wine with dinner raises my morning fasting glucose" - "I need to walk after any meal with rice" - "Eating eggs for breakfast keeps me stable until lunch" - "Evening carbs disrupt my sleep and glucose"

**Practical Application**: Write down your top 5-10 food rules based on your CGM data. These become your personalized weight loss guidelines—

far more effective than following generic diet advice.

# Chapter 6: Common CGM Insights for Weight Loss

One of the first things the CGM taught me was that the foods I'd trusted most were the ones doing the most damage. I'd been starting every morning with what I thought was a healthy breakfast, and watching my glucose hit 165 before 9 AM. This chapter is about those surprises — the patterns that show up for nearly everyone once they start looking at real data rather than nutrition labels and conventional wisdom.

## Breakfast Revelations

Many people discover that their "healthy" breakfast is sabotaging their entire day. Common culprits:

Instant oatmeal is one of the most common surprises — despite its health-food reputation, the processing that makes it instant also strips away the structural fiber that slows glucose absorption. Steel-cut oats from the same grain behave very differently. Fruit smoothies are another trap: blending destroys the cellular structure of fruit, so the glucose from three blended bananas hits your bloodstream far faster than three whole bananas would. Toast and jam — even whole grain toast — is essentially a high-carbohydrate delivery system with minimal protein or fat to slow it down. Add eggs or nut butter and watch what happens to the curve. Even breakfast cereals marketed with health claims will often send your glucose to 150 or above before 8 AM, setting off a chain of insulin and cravings that follows you through the entire morning.

**Fruit Smoothies**: Blending destroys fiber structure and creates rapid glucose spikes. Whole fruit is far better.

**Toast and Jam**: Pure carbohydrate bomb. Add eggs or nut butter.

**Breakfast Cereal**: Even "healthy" cereals often spike glucose dramatically. Test carefully.

**The Solution**: A protein-rich breakfast (eggs, Greek yogurt, protein smoothie with minimal fruit) often keeps glucose stable for hours and reduces total daily hunger.

**The Sandwich Problem**

Bread is one of the most reliable glucose spikers in the modern diet, and this includes whole wheat. The issue isn't just the flour — it's the density of carbohydrate with very little fat or protein to buffer it. Open-faced sandwiches using a single slice reduce the carbohydrate load by half. Lettuce wraps eliminate it almost entirely while keeping everything you want in the sandwich. Many people find that eating the sandwich filling — the protein, cheese, avocado, vegetables — without the bread produces a completely flat glucose line and feels just as satisfying.

**Solutions**: - Open-faced sandwiches (one slice) - Lettuce wraps - Lower-carb bread alternatives - Eat the sandwich filling without bread - If you do eat sandwiches, pair with protein, fat, and vegetables and consider a post-meal walk

**The Dinner Dilemma**

Many people save their largest meal for dinner, but CGM data often shows this is when we're most insulin resistant. Large evening meals, especially with carbohydrates, can:

- Cause prolonged glucose elevation
- Disrupt sleep quality
- Elevate morning fasting glucose
- Increase next-day insulin resistance

**The Solution**: Consider making lunch your largest meal or at least front-loading your carbohydrates earlier in the day.

### Snacking Patterns

Frequent snacking creates a problem that the scale doesn't show you, but your CGM will. Even when individual snacks don't cause dramatic spikes, each one triggers an insulin response that keeps your body in storage mode rather than burning mode. The effect compounds across a day: a mid-morning snack, a mid-afternoon snack, a handful of something before dinner — and insulin has been elevated almost continuously from breakfast to bed, with very little window for fat burning. Most people find that eating satisfying, well-composed meals without snacking between them creates the longest periods of low insulin and the most productive fat-burning windows.

**What Often Happens**: - Snack at 10 AM: glucose rises slightly, insulin rises - Returns to baseline by noon - Lunch at 12 PM: glucose and insulin rise again - Snack at 3 PM: glucose rises again before fully recovering - Dinner at 7 PM: another rise - Evening snack at 9 PM: yet another rise

Insulin is elevated almost continuously, blocking fat burning all day.

**The Solution**: Many people find that eating satisfying meals without snacking allows for periods of lower insulin and better fat burning. Your CGM will show when you've truly returned to baseline.

**The Alcohol Effect**

Alcohol's effects on glucose are more complicated than most people expect. It often lowers glucose initially — especially on an empty stomach — because the liver prioritizes metabolizing the alcohol over releasing stored glucose. But this is frequently followed by a rebound elevation several hours later as the liver overcorrects. The next morning's fasting glucose is often meaningfully higher after an evening of drinking, and the body's response to breakfast that day tends to be blunted. Sleep quality also suffers, which compounds the metabolic cost. None of this means abstinence is required — it means your CGM can show you your specific response pattern and help you make informed decisions about timing and quantity.

- May lower glucose initially (especially on an empty stomach)
- Often followed by rebound elevation as the liver releases stored glucose
- Frequently raises fasting glucose the next morning

- Impairs the body's response to the next meal
- Disrupts sleep, which further impairs glucose control

**Practical Application**: Test your typical alcoholic drinks and see the full 24-hour impact, including next-day effects.

**Exercise Insights**

Different types of exercise affect glucose differently:

**Aerobic Exercise**: Usually lowers glucose during and after the activity. Great for blunting a post-meal spike.

**High-Intensity Interval Training (HIIT)**: May raise glucose during exercise due to stress hormone release but improves insulin sensitivity for hours afterward.

**Strength Training**: Typically raises glucose slightly during the workout but dramatically improves glucose disposal for 24-48 hours.

**Timing Matters**: Exercise before a meal often allows you to handle more carbohydrates. Exercise after a meal blunts the spike.

**The "Health Food" Trap**

Perhaps the most liberating thing the CGM does is render marketing irrelevant. Granola and granola bars, most energy and protein bars, dried fruit, fruit juice including green juices, agave and other "natural" sweeteners, and many gluten-free products are all capable of causing significant glucose spikes despite the health language on their packaging. The CGM doesn't read labels. It reads what happens in your blood. That's not a judgement of these foods — it's permission to stop feeling virtuous about them if your data tells you otherwise.

- Granola and granola bars
- Most "energy" or "protein" bars
- Dried fruit
- Fruit juice and "green" juices
- Agave nectar and other "natural" sweeteners
- Many gluten-free products (often high in refined starch)

Your CGM doesn't care about marketing claims—it shows you the actual metabolic impact.

> *Your CGM is one of the most empowering tools you can bring to a conversation with your doctor or dietitian. Rather than relying on food labels or general guidelines, you arrive with your own data — your specific responses to specific foods. Nutrition science continues to evolve, and what works for one person may not work for another. The CGM bridges that gap beautifully, giving you and your healthcare provider a*

*shared, objective starting point for making decisions that are truly personalized to you.* → ***See: A Note on Evidence, Independence, and Medication***

# Chapter 7: Building Your CGM-Based Weight Loss Plan

After the first two weeks of just observing, I needed a structure — a way to turn all those data points into a deliberate plan. What I found was that the plan didn't need to be complicated; it just needed to evolve in stages. First understand your baseline, then experiment, then build habits around what works. This chapter maps out that progression, so you know exactly where you are in the process and what to focus on next.

### Phase 1: The 2-Week Assessment (Weeks 1-2)

**Goals**: - Establish baseline glucose patterns - Identify problem foods and meals - Test key variables (timing, sequencing, movement) - Begin building your personal food database

**Daily Actions**: - Wear your CGM continuously - Log all food, sleep, exercise, and stress - Review data each evening - Take screenshots of interesting patterns - Begin experimenting with modifications

**End of Phase 1**: You should have clear insights into your current patterns and several proven strategies for improving glucose control.

**Phase 2: Implementation (Weeks 3-6)**

**Goals**: - Apply your learnings consistently - Refine your personal food rules - Build new habits around timing, sequencing, and movement - Track weight loss progress

**Daily Actions**: - Follow your personalized food rules - Apply vegetable-first sequencing to meals - Take post-meal walks, especially after higher-carb meals - Prioritize sleep and stress management - Continue logging and reviewing data

**Expected Results**: Most people see: - More stable glucose throughout the day - Reduced hunger and cravings - better energy levels - Improved sleep - Initial weight loss (2-6 pounds depending on starting weight)

**Phase 3: Optimization (Weeks 7-12)**

**Goals**: - Fine-tune your approach - Test edge cases and special situations - Develop strategies for dining out, travel, celebrations - Build sustainable long-term habits

**Daily Actions**: - Continue proven strategies - Experiment with reintroducing challenging foods in new contexts - Test different carbohydrate thresholds - Practice your protocols in varied situations - Track progress and adjust as needed

**Expected Results**: - Continued steady weight loss (1-2 pounds per week) - Strong metabolic improvements - Confident understanding of your glucose responses - Sustainable habits that don't feel restrictive

**Phase 4: Independence (Month 4+)**

**Goals**: - Transition to intermittent CGM use - Maintain weight loss - Continue optimization - Integrate learnings permanently

**Approach**: Many people don't need to wear a CGM continuously long-term. After several months, you've built a deep understanding of your responses. Consider:

- Wearing a CGM 1-2 weeks per month to stay calibrated
- Using it when testing new foods or strategies
- Returning to it during times of stress or travel
- Periodic check-ins to prevent habit drift

**Long-term Success**: The goal is to internalize the principles so deeply that you instinctively know how to keep your glucose stable and weight off, even without continuous monitoring.

## Chapter 8: Troubleshooting Common Challenges

There were weeks when the data confused me. I'd done everything right and my glucose was still spiking. Or the weight had stalled despite stable readings. These plateaus and puzzles are normal — they're not signs that the approach is failing, they're signs that your body is asking a more specific question. This chapter answers the questions I kept running into, and the ones I hear most often from others who've been through this process.

### "My glucose still spikes even when I follow the rules"

**Possible Causes**: - Insufficient protein or fat with carbohydrates - Portion sizes too large - Timing issues (eating too late in the day) - High stress or poor sleep affecting insulin sensitivity - Individual intolerance to specific foods - Medical conditions affecting metabolism

**Solutions**: - Reduce carbohydrate portions further - Increase protein and healthy fats - Move meals earlier in the day - Address sleep and stress -

Consider eliminating specific trigger foods - Consult with a healthcare provider

**"I'm not losing weight despite stable glucose"**

**Possible Causes**: - Eating too many calories overall (even stable glucose requires a calorie deficit for weight loss) - Not enough physical activity - Metabolic adaptation from previous dieting - Hormonal issues (thyroid, cortisol, sex hormones) - Insufficient sleep - Medications that affect weight **Solutions**: - Track total calorie intake for a week - Increase daily movement and exercise - Ensure adequate protein intake (supports satiety and muscle) - Prioritize sleep optimization - Consider comprehensive metabolic testing - Consult with a healthcare provider

**"My morning fasting glucose is high"**

**Dawn Phenomenon Causes**: - Normal cortisol rise in early morning - Poor sleep quality - Late-night eating - Chronic stress - Insufficient physical activity

**Solutions**: - Stop eating 3 hours before bed - Take an evening walk - Practice stress reduction - Ensure 7-9 hours of quality sleep - Consider morning exercise to improve insulin sensitivity - Test bedtime protein snacks (helps some people)

**"I can't afford continuous CGM use"**

**Cost-Effective Strategies**: - Use CGM for 2-4 weeks initially to gather key insights - Wear it intermittently (1 week per month) to stay calibrated - Focus on building habits during CGM periods that you maintain between uses - Share learnings with friends who might split costs - Look for cheaper alternatives or programs offering subsidized CGMs **Non-CGM Alternatives**: - Track energy levels, hunger, and cravings after meals as proxies for glucose stability - Use occasional finger-stick glucose testing around meals - Follow proven principles even without monitoring

**"My CGM readings seem inaccurate"**

**Common Issues**: - Sensor placement on muscle or areas with poor circulation - Compression of sensor during sleep - Sensor at beginning or end of its lifespan - Dehydration - Interference from certain medications (like acetaminophen)

**Solutions**: - Ensure proper sensor placement (back of upper arm usually best) - Avoid sleeping on the sensor - Stay well hydrated - Confirm suspicious readings with finger-stick test - Contact manufacturer if persistent issues

# Chapter 9: Beyond Weight Loss - Long-Term Metabolic Health

About two months in, something shifted that had nothing to do with the scale. My energy was steadier, my thinking was clearer, and a fog I'd gotten so used to I'd stopped noticing it had quietly lifted. Weight loss had been the goal, but metabolic health turned out to be the prize. This chapter is about what you're building when you stabilize your glucose — and why the benefits compound long after the weight comes off.

## Metabolic Syndrome Reversal

Metabolic syndrome is a cluster of conditions (high blood pressure, high blood sugar, excess abdominal fat, abnormal cholesterol) that increase risk of heart disease, stroke, and diabetes. CGM-guided eating can help support improvements in these markers.

*Metabolic syndrome is a serious medical condition. While lifestyle changes including those supported by CGM data can meaningfully improve these markers, do not attempt to self-manage metabolic syndrome without healthcare provider involvement. High blood pressure, elevated cholesterol, and pre-diabetic glucose levels require medical monitoring. Use this book's strategies as a complement to — not a replacement for — professional medical care.*

**Improvements You Might See**: - Lower fasting glucose and HbA1c - Improved insulin sensitivity - better cholesterol ratios - Reduced blood pressure - Decreased waist circumference - Reduced inflammation markers

**Tracking Progress**: Work with your doctor to monitor these markers every 3-6 months as you implement CGM-based strategies.

**Preventing Type 2 Diabetes**

If you have prediabetes (fasting glucose 100-125 mg/dL or HbA1c 5.7-6.4%), a CGM can be invaluable for preventing progression to type 2 diabetes.

**Key Strategies**: - Keep post-meal glucose under 140 mg/dL consistently - Minimize time above 120 mg/dL - Reduce glucose variability - Build muscle through strength training - Lose 5-10% of body weight if overweight

Studies show these strategies can reduce diabetes risk by over 50%. [Diabetes Prevention Program Research Group, 2002, NEJM; Knowler et al., 2002]

*Important: If you have prediabetes or are at high risk for Type 2 diabetes, do not attempt to manage this condition through CGM-guided lifestyle changes alone without medical supervision. Medically supervised programs such as the CDC-recognized Diabetes Prevention Program (DPP) have the strongest evidence base. Please consult your healthcare provider or a certified diabetes educator for personalized guidance.*

> *A note if you are using or considering GLP-1 medications : the lifestyle strategies in this book work beautifully alongside these treatments. GLP-1 therapies and CGM-guided habits engage many of the same metabolic pathways — better glucose stability, reduced appetite, improved insulin sensitivity — and the combination is genuinely powerful. If you are on GLP-1 medication, please continue under your doctor's guidance. The habits in this book will support and reinforce everything your treatment is working toward. Always discuss any changes to your health routine with your physician first.* → ***See: A Note on Evidence, Independence, and Medication***

## Cognitive Function and Brain Health

Emerging research links glucose variability to cognitive decline and Alzheimer's disease. Stable glucose supports:

- Better focus and concentration
- Improved memory

- Enhanced mood stability
- Reduced brain fog
- Potential support for long-term brain health (research ongoing)

**Longevity and Health span**

Lower average glucose and reduced glucose variability are associated with:

- Decreased inflammation
- Reduced oxidative stress
- Better cellular energy production
- Associations with healthy ageing markers (observational data)
- Reduced risk of chronic diseases

The metabolic optimization you achieve for weight loss also supports longevity and quality of life as you age.

**Athletic Performance**

Even if not an athlete, the glucose stability you develop improves:

- Sustained energy during physical activity
- Faster recovery
- Better body composition
- Enhanced endurance
- Improved strength gains

Many athletes now use CGMs to optimize nutrition timing around training.

# Chapter 10: Maintaining Your Success

The morning, I took off my last CGM sensor, I was nervous. The device had become my feedback loop, my teacher, my accountability partner. But what I realized over the weeks that followed was that the sensor had done its job: I'd internalized what it taught me. I no longer needed to check the graph after every meal because I already knew, from feel and from habit, what my body's answer would be. That's the goal of this final chapter — not dependence on the tool, but the wisdom it leaves behind.

## Building Lasting Habits

The behaviors that help you lose weight with a CGM need to become permanent habits for lasting success:

**The Core Habits**: 1. Protein-rich breakfast 2. Vegetable-first eating sequence 3. Post-meal movement (especially after larger meals) 4. Eating window aligned with circadian rhythm 5. Prioritizing sleep and stress management 6. Staying hydrated 7. Regular physical activity

**Habit Stacking**: Link new behaviors to existing routines: - "After I make coffee, I'll prepare my protein breakfast" - "Before I eat lunch, I'll eat my salad" - "After dinner is cleared, I'll take my walk"

**Periodic CGM Check-ins**

Even after initial weight loss, consider wearing a CGM periodically:

**Quarterly Reviews** (wear for 1-2 weeks): - Verify your habits are still effective - Test new foods or strategies - Recalibrate your instincts - Catch any habit drift early

**Trigger Events**: Wear a CGM during: - Times of increased stress - Travel or routine disruption - Weight loss plateaus - After regaining a few pounds - When trying significant diet changes

**Navigating Social Situations**

Real life includes restaurants, holidays, and celebrations. Your CGM experience provides tools to handle these:

**Restaurant Strategies**: - Review menus in advance - Order protein-and-vegetable-focused meals - Ask for substitutions (vegetables instead of rice) - Share desserts or skip them - Take a walk after the meal

**Holiday Approaches**: - Eat well before events so you're not starving - Focus on protein and vegetables first - Choose your indulgences deliberately - Stay active - Return to your regular routine immediately after

**The 80/20 Rule**: If your glucose is stable 80% of the time, you can afford some flexibility 20% of the time without derailing your progress.

**Handling Plateaus**

Weight loss plateaus are normal. When they occur:

**Review Your Data**: - Has your glucose stability slipped? - Are portions creeping up? - Has stress or sleep quality declined? - Are you moving less?

**Strategies to Break Plateaus**: - Return to strict CGM monitoring for 1-2 weeks - Reduce carbohydrates temporarily - Increase protein intake - Add strength training - Implement intermittent fasting - Address sleep or stress issues

**Remember**: Sometimes plateaus represent metabolic adaptation to your new weight. Patience and consistency matter more than dramatic changes.

### Dealing with Setbacks

Everyone experiences setbacks. The difference is in how you respond:

**When You Regain a Few Pounds**:

1. Put your CGM back on
2. Review what changed in your habits
3. Recommit to your core principles
4. Don't wait—act immediately
5. Be kind to yourself while staying accountable

**Avoiding All-or-Nothing Thinking**: One high-glucose meal doesn't ruin your progress. Get back on track with your next meal. Consistency over time matters far more than perfection.

## Chapter 11: Success Stories and Practical Examples

The patterns I've described throughout this book don't just appear in my data – they show up again in people with completely different bodies, diets, and starting points. What the following stories illustrate isn't that everyone's journey looks the same; it's that the underlying mechanism is remarkably consistent. When you stop chasing a generic diet and start responding to your own data, the results tend to follow.

**Important Note**: The following stories are composite examples created for illustrative purposes, drawing from common patterns and experiences reported in CGM weight loss research and user communities. They are not based on specific real individuals but rather represent typical scenarios and outcomes that many people experience when using CGM technology for weight loss. Individual results will vary based on numerous factors including genetics, adherence, starting metabolic health, and lifestyle factors.

**Sarah's Story: Breaking the Bread Habit**

Sarah, a composite example representing a common pattern, was 42 and had struggled with weight for years despite eating what she considered a healthy diet. When she started using a CGM, she discovered that her morning toast routine was spiking her glucose to 165 mg/dL, followed by a crash that left her ravenous by mid-morning.

**What Changed**: - Switched to eggs and avocado for breakfast - Glucose stayed stable around 95 mg/dL - No mid-morning cravings - Lost 23 pounds in 4 months

**Key Insight**: "I thought I was doing everything right. The CGM showed me that 'healthy whole grain toast' was setting me up to fail every single day."

**Michael's Story: The Evening Carb Discovery**

Michael, representing a pattern commonly seen in middle-aged men, was 55 and exercised regularly but couldn't lose his last 20 pounds. His CGM revealed that dinner was his problem meal—large pasta portions at 8 PM were keeping his glucose elevated until midnight and raising his fasting glucose the next morning.

**What Changed**: - Moved dinner to 6 PM - Replaced pasta with cauliflower rice and more protein - Added an after-dinner walk - Glucose returned to baseline by 9 PM - Morning fasting glucose dropped from 105 to 88 mg/dL - Lost 18 pounds in 3 months

**Key Insight**: "Timing was everything. The same meal earlier in the day had half the glucose impact."

**Jennifer's Story: The Stress Connection**

Jennifer, an illustrative example of stress-related glucose issues, was 38 and ate impeccably but couldn't understand why her weight loss had stalled. Her CGM revealed that work stress was spiking her glucose to 130-140 mg/dL during afternoon meetings—without eating anything.

**What Changed**: - Implemented 5-minute breathing exercises before stressful meetings - Started taking short walks during breaks - Improved sleep hygiene to reduce overall stress - Stress-related spikes decreased significantly - Weight loss resumed

**Key Insight**: "I had no idea my body was responding to stress the same way it responds to sugar. Managing stress became as important as managing my diet."

**David's Story: The Personalized Approach**

David, representing the importance of individual metabolic variation, was 48 and discovered through his CGM that he had unusual responses to foods. He could eat white rice with minimal spike, but oatmeal sent his glucose soaring. Bananas were fine, but apples caused problems.

**What Changed**: - Built his diet around his personal responses rather than generic "healthy food" lists - Kept detailed notes on his best and worst foods - Used food sequencing and post-meal walks for foods that moderately spiked him - Lost

31 pounds and felt he finally understood his metabolism

**Key Insight**: "Every diet I tried before was based on what worked for other people. This was the first time I had a plan designed specifically for my body."

## Conclusion: Your Metabolic Journey

Using a CGM for weight loss isn't just about the number on the scale—it's about understanding your unique metabolism and building a sustainable relationship with food based on data rather than guesswork.

The insights you gain transcend any specific diet or trend. You learn:

- **How your individual body responds** to different foods, timing, and contexts
- **What genuine metabolic health feels like**—stable energy, minimal cravings, good sleep
- **The power of personalization** over one-size-fits-all approaches
- **How to make informed choices** rather than following rigid rules

This knowledge is permanent. Even if you stop wearing a CGM daily, you've built an intuitive understanding of how to keep your glucose stable and your metabolism healthy.

The weight you lose this way tends to stay off because you haven't followed an unsustainable diet—you've discovered how your body works and built habits around that reality.

**Your Next Steps**

1. **Obtain a CGM**: The author used Lingo by Abbott (hellolingo.com). To find options in your region, search "CGM for wellness" in your local search engine.
2. **Commit to Learning**: Give yourself at least 4-6 weeks of consistent monitoring and experimentation
3. **Track Systematically**: Log food, exercise, sleep, and stress alongside your glucose data
4. **Stay Curious**: Approach this as a scientific exploration of your unique metabolism
5. **Be Patient**: Metabolic improvements and weight loss take time, but the knowledge you gain is invaluable
6. **Share Your Journey**: Consider connecting with others using CGMs for mutual support and insights

## Final Thoughts

For too long, weight loss has been framed as a battle of willpower against hunger. But hunger is often a symptom of unstable glucose, and willpower is finite.

A CGM gives you a different path—one based on understanding cause and effect in your own body. When you see in real-time how different foods affect your glucose, cravings, and energy, making healthy choices becomes easier and more intuitive.

This is personalized nutrition in its truest form. Not a celebrity's meal plan or a bestselling diet book, but your body's actual metabolic responses, revealed in unprecedented detail.

The glucose code has always been there, running silently in the background of your metabolism. Now you can read it, understand it, and use it to finally achieve the sustainable weight loss and vibrant health you deserve.

Your journey begins with a single sensor and one simple question: "How does my body respond to this?"

The answers will transform everything.

# Appendix A: CGM Quick Reference Guide

## Getting Started Checklist

- Order CGM from chosen provider
- Download associated app
- Set up food logging system
- Establish baseline metrics (weight, measurements, photos)
- Read user manual for sensor application
- Plan 2-week baseline eating period
- Set up data review routine

## Daily Monitoring Protocol

- Check morning fasting glucose
- Log all meals with timing
- Note energy and hunger levels post-meal
- Record exercise, sleep quality, stress
- Review evening glucose patterns
- Screenshot interesting data
- Adjust next day's plan based on insights

## Target Ranges (Non-Diabetic Adults)

- Fasting glucose: 70-100 mg/dL
- Post-meal peak: <140 mg/dL (optimal <110 mg/dL)
- Time in range (70-120 mg/dL): >90%
- Average daily glucose: 90-100 mg/dL
- Standard deviation: <15-20 mg/dL

**Food Testing Template**

**Food being tested**: ________________

**Portion size**: ________________

**Time consumed**: ________________

**Baseline glucose**: ________________

**Peak glucose**: ________________

**Time to peak**: ________________

**Time to return to baseline**: ________________

**Spike magnitude**: ________________

**How I felt**: ________________

**Would eat again?** ________________

# Appendix B: Walking Alternatives

## 10 Direct Walking Alternatives

### 1. Household Chores (30 minutes = 30 min walking)

- Vacuuming, mopping, washing dishes by hand
- Laundry (folding, putting away)
- Tidying and organizing
- Any active cleaning
- Bonus: Gets chores done while lowering glucose!

**2. Stair Climbing (10-15 minutes = 30 min walking)**

- Walk up and down stairs in your home or building
- 2-3x MORE effective than walking
- Quick and efficient
- Caution: Start slow if you're not used to it

**3. Stationary Bike or Cycling (20-25 minutes = 30 min walking)**

- Stationary bike at home or gym
- Recumbent bike (easier on joints)
- Under-desk pedal exerciser
- Keep resistance LOW for post-meal use
- Perfect for watching TV or reading

**4. Swimming or Water Walking (15-20 minutes = 30 min walking)**

- Leisure swimming
- Water walking in pool
- Aqua aerobics (light)
- Zero impact on joints
- Often MORE effective than walking

**5. Dancing (20-25 minutes = 30 min walking)**

- Kitchen dance party to your favorite music
- Any style—just move!
- Fun and stress-relieving
- Equivalent or better glucose-lowering effect

**6. Yard Work (20 minutes = 30 min walking)**

- Raking leaves, gardening, weeding
- Mowing lawn, trimming hedges
- Watering plants
- Often BETTER than walking for glucose control
- Bonus: Fresh air and productive

**7. Standing Desk Work (30-45 minutes = 30 min walking)**

- Stand while working at computer
- Stand during phone calls
- Shift weight, do calf raises occasionally
- 60-70% as effective as walking
- Perfect for work-from-home situations

### 8. Playing with Kids or Pets (20-30 minutes)

• Active play with children

• Playing with or walking dog

• Active games

• Equivalent to walking

• Bonus: Quality time!

### 9. Resistance Band Exercises (15-20 minutes = 30 min walking)

• Light resistance band movements

• Bicep curls, shoulder presses, squats with band

• Often BETTER than walking

• Builds muscle = better long-term glucose control

• Perfect for small spaces

### 10. Active Errands (30 minutes)

• Grocery shopping (walking around store)

• Mall walking

• Running errands on foot

• Equivalent to walking

• Bonus: Productive!

## Cold Weather & Bad Weather Solutions

When it's too cold, icy, or stormy to walk outside:

- Mall walking (indoors, climate-controlled)
- Indoor track at gym or community center
- Treadmill at home or gym
- Stair climbing in your building
- Walking in place while watching TV
- YouTube walking videos (follow along at home)
- Household chores (always available!)
- Dancing to music in your living room

### For Mobility Issues or Injuries

If you have mobility limitations, injuries, or can't walk:

- Seated pedal exerciser (under-desk pedals)
- Chair exercises or chair yoga
- Arm movements and upper body exercises
- Swimming or water walking (no joint stress)
- Recumbent bike (seated, back supported)
- Gentle seated stretching

**Key:** ANY movement helps. Even 10 minutes is better than zero!

## Solutions for Office Workers

Can't leave your desk for 30 minutes after meals?

• Under-desk pedal exerciser (pedal while working)

• Standing desk (stand for 45 minutes after lunch)

• Micro-movements: Stand up every 10 min, do 20 squats, walk to water cooler

• Take stairs to different floor a few times

• Walk during phone calls

• Lunch walk: Eat quickly (15 min), walk remaining 45 min

## The Key Principle

**The goal is movement that uses your muscles to lower glucose after meals.** It doesn't have to be walking.

I used walking because it was simple and accessible for me. You should use whatever movement fits YOUR life, YOUR body, and YOUR circumstances.

Some alternatives (like stair climbing or resistance training) are actually MORE effective than walking in less time. Some (like chores or errands) accomplish two goals at once. Some (like dancing or playing with kids) are more fun.

**The best movement is the one you'll do consistently.**

Experiment with different options. Use your CGM to see what works best for YOUR body. Mix and match based on weather, schedule, and mood.

Your journey is YOUR journey. Make it work for you.

### Quick Reference: Time Equivalents

Here's how other activities compare to 30 minutes of walking:

- 10-15 min stair climbing = 30 min walking
- 15-20 min swimming = 30 min walking
- 15-20 min resistance training = 30 min walking
- 20-25 min cycling = 30 min walking
- 20-25 min dancing = 30 min walking
- 20 min yard work = 30 min walking
- 30 min chores = 30 min walking
- 30 min active errands = 30 min walking
- 45 min standing desk work = 30 min walking

Remember: Any movement is better than no movement. If you can only do 10 minutes, do 10 minutes. Something is always better than nothing when it comes to lowering post-meal glucose.

# Appendix C: Recommended Resources

## Reference Data: Healthy Weight Ranges

Understanding where you currently stand and setting realistic goals is important for your weight loss journey. Below are evidence-based reference ranges and tools to help you assess your status and track progress.

*Body Mass Index (BMI) Reference Ranges*

BMI is calculated as: **Weight (kg) / Height (m)²** or **Weight (lbs) / Height (inches)² × 703**

**Standard BMI Categories (Adults 20+)**:

- **Underweight**: BMI less than 18.5
- **Normal weight**: BMI 18.5-24.9
- **Overweight**: BMI 25.0-29.9
- **Obesity Class I**: BMI 30.0-34.9
- **Obesity Class II**: BMI 35.0-39.9
- **Obesity Class III**: BMI 40.0 or higher

**Important Note**: BMI is a screening tool and has limitations. It doesn't distinguish between muscle and fat, doesn't account for body composition, and may not be accurate for athletes, older adults, or certain ethnic groups. Use it as one data point among many, not as the definitive measure of health.

*Healthy Weight Ranges by Height (Adults)*

These ranges represent the "normal" BMI category (18.5-24.9) for different heights:

**For Imperial Measurements (feet/inches and pounds)**:

| Height | Healthy Weight Range (BMI 18.5-24.9) |
|---|---|
| 4'10" (58") | 91-115 lbs |
| 4'11" (59") | 94-119 lbs |
| 5'0" (60") | 97-123 lbs |
| 5'1" (61") | 100-127 lbs |
| 5'2" (62") | 104-131 lbs |
| 5'3" (63") | 107-135 lbs |
| 5'4" (64") | 110-140 lbs |
| 5'5" (65") | 114-144 lbs |
| 5'6" (66") | 118-148 lbs |
| 5'7" (67") | 121-153 lbs |
| 5'8" (68") | 125-158 lbs |
| 5'9" (69") | 128-162 lbs |
| 5'10" (70") | 132-167 lbs |

| Height | Healthy Weight Range (BMI 18.5-24.9) |
|---|---|
| 5'11" (71") | 136-172 lbs |
| 6'0" (72") | 140-177 lbs |
| 6'1" (73") | 144-182 lbs |
| 6'2" (74") | 148-186 lbs |
| 6'3" (75") | 152-192 lbs |
| 6'4" (76") | 156-197 lbs |

**For Metric Measurements (centimeters and kilograms)**:

| Height | Healthy Weight Range (BMI 18.5-24.9) |
|---|---|
| 147 cm | 41-52 kg |
| 150 cm | 42-54 kg |
| 152 cm | 43-55 kg |
| 155 cm | 44-57 kg |
| 157 cm | 46-58 kg |
| 160 cm | 47-60 kg |
| 163 cm | 49-62 kg |
| 165 cm | 50-64 kg |
| 168 cm | 52-66 kg |
| 170 cm | 53-67 kg |
| 173 cm | 55-70 kg |
| 175 cm | 57-72 kg |
| 178 cm | 59-74 kg |
| 180 cm | 60-76 kg |
| 183 cm | 62-78 kg |

| Height | Healthy Weight Range (BMI 18.5-24.9) |
|---|---|
| 185 cm | 63-80 kg |
| 188 cm | 65-83 kg |
| 191 cm | 67-85 kg |
| 193 cm | 69-87 kg |

*Age-Related Considerations*

**Adults Under 40**: Use standard BMI ranges as listed above

**Adults 40-60**: - Metabolism naturally slows with age - Muscle mass tends to decrease (sarcopenia) - BMI ranges remain the same, but body composition matters more - Focus on maintaining muscle through strength training

**Adults 60+**: - Some research suggests slightly higher BMI (up to 27) may be protective in older adults - Muscle mass and functional fitness become more important than absolute weight - Unintentional weight loss is concerning and should be evaluated by a doctor - Maintain strength and mobility as primary health markers

**Note**: These are general guidelines. Always consult with a healthcare provider for personalized recommendations, especially if you're over 60 or have specific health conditions.

*Waist Circumference: An Important Additional Metric*

Waist circumference measures abdominal fat and is a strong predictor of metabolic disease risk, often more accurate than BMI alone.

**Measure at the narrowest point of your waist, usually just above the belly button**

**Health Risk by Waist Circumference**:

**Target**: Waist circumference < 0.5 × Height

-https://www.nhlbi.nih.gov/health/heart-healthy-living/healthy-weight

Reducing waist circumference is a key goal for metabolic health, even if overall weight loss is modest.

*Waist-to-Height Ratio*

A newer, simpler metric: Your waist circumference should be less than half your height.

**Target**: Waist circumference < 0.5 × Height

**Examples**: - Height 5'8" (68 inches): Waist should be less than 34 inches - Height 6'0" (72 inches): Waist should be less than 36 inches - Height 170 cm: Waist should be less than 85 cm - Height 180 cm: Waist should be less than 90 cm

https://www.nhs.uk/health-assessment-tools/calculate-your-waist-to-height-ratio

**Comprehensive Health Risk Assessment**:

*Online Calculators and Health Assessment Tools*

**BMI Calculators**:

- **CDC BMI Calculator**: https://www.cdc.gov/bmi/adult-calculator/index.html - Official CDC tool, easy to use, provides category classification

- **NIH BMI Calculator**: https://www.nhlbi.nih.gov/health/educational/lose_wt/BMI/bmicalc.htm - National Heart, Lung, and Blood Institute calculator with additional resources

**Comprehensive Health Risk Assessment**:

- **CDC WISEWOMAN**: https://www.cdc.gov/wisewoman/ - cardiovascular disease risk screening and lifestyle programs

- **AHA Heart Health Assessment**: https://www.heart.org/en/healthy-living - American Heart Association resources for cardiovascular health

**Waist-to-Height Ratio Information**:

- **British Nutrition Foundation**: https://www.nutrition.org.uk/ - Includes waist-to-height ratio information and assessment tools

**Body Fat Percentage Calculators** (estimates based on measurements): - **Navy Body Fat Calculator**: https://www.calculator.net/body-fat-calculator.html

- Uses circumference measurements to estimate body fat percentage - **YMCA Body Fat Calculator**: Available through fitness centers and online tools

**Metabolic Health Screening**:

- **ADA Prediabetes Risk Test**: https://diabetes.org/risk-test - American Diabetes Association screening tool for diabetes risk (takes 1 minute) - **CDC Diabetes Prevention Program**: https://www.cdc.gov/diabetes/prevention/ - Resources for preventing type 2 diabetes

**Nutrition and Weight Management Resources**: - **USDA MyPlate**: https://www.myplate.gov/ - Government nutrition guidance and meal planning tools - **Academy of Nutrition and Dietetics**: https://www.eatright.org/ - Find registered dietitians and evidence-based nutrition information - **NIH Weight Control Information Network**: https://www.niddk.nih.gov/health-information/weight-management - Comprehensive weight management resources from National Institutes of Health

**Physical Activity Guidelines**:

- **CDC Physical Activity Guidelines**: https://www.cdc.gov/physicalactivity/basics/adults/index.htm - Official recommendations for adult physical activity

- **American College of Sports Medicine**: https://www.acsm.org/ - Exercise prescription guidelines and fitness resources

**Sleep Resources**:

- **National Sleep Foundation**: https://www.sleepfoundation.org/ - Evidence-based sleep information and tips for better sleep

- **CDC Sleep and Sleep Disorders**: https://www.cdc.gov/sleep/ - Public health perspective on sleep health

**Mental Health and Stress Management**:

- **National Alliance on Mental Illness (NAMI)**: https://www.nami.org/ - Mental health resources and support

- **Anxiety & Depression Association of America**: https://adaa.org/ - Resources for managing anxiety and depression
- **Headspace**: https://www.headspace.com/ (meditation app)
- **Calm**: https://www.calm.com/ (meditation and sleep app)

`Setting Your Personal Weight Loss Goal`

**Conservative Goal**: - Lose 5-10% of your current body weight - Example: If you weigh 200 lbs, aim for 10-20 lbs initially

- This amount produces significant metabolic improvements

**Moderate Goal**: - Reach the upper end of the healthy BMI range (BMI of 24-25) - Reduces disease risk while being achievable for most people

**Optimal Goal**: - Reach the middle of the healthy BMI range (BMI of 21-23) - Often the weight at which people feel and function best - May take longer to achieve but offers maximum health benefits

**Realistic Timeline**:

- **Healthy weight loss rate**: 1-2 pounds per week (0.5-1 kg)
- **To lose 20 pounds**: 10-20 weeks (2.5-5 months)

- **To lose 50 pounds**: 25-50 weeks (6-12 months)
- **To lose 100 pounds**: 50-100 weeks (12-24 months)

Remember: Slow, steady weight loss is more sustainable and more likely to be maintained long-term than rapid weight loss.

*Important Reminders*

1. **These are population averages, not personal prescriptions**: Your optimal weight depends on many factors including genetics, muscle mass, bone density, age, and overall health status.
2. **Metabolic health matters more than weight alone**: Someone at a higher BMI with excellent glucose control, good cardiovascular fitness, and healthy blood pressure may be healthier than someone at a "normal" BMI with metabolic dysfunction.
3. **Your CGM data is more important than the scale**: Focus on improving your glucose patterns, reducing insulin resistance, and building healthy behaviors. The weight will follow.
4. **Consult healthcare professionals**: Before starting any weight loss program,

especially if you have significant weight to lose or existing health conditions, work with your doctor, and consider consulting a registered dietitian.

5. **Body composition changes matter**: You may lose fat while gaining muscle, especially if doing strength training. The scale might not move much, but your body composition, health markers, and how you feel are improving dramatically.

## CGM Providers

- **Lingo** by Abbott (used by the author): hellolingo.com

  To find CGM options in your region, search "CGM for weight loss" or "continuous glucose monitor wellness" in your local search engine. Availability, pricing, and whether a prescription is required varies by country and region.

## Additional Reading

- "The Glucose Revolution" by Jessie Inchauspé
- "Good Energy" by Dr. Casey Means
- "Why We Get Sick" by Dr. Benjamin Bikman

- Research from Weizmann Institute on personalized nutrition

**Online Communities**

- CGM user forums and subreddits
- Metabolic health discussion groups
- Provider-specific community platforms

## Appendix D: Acronyms

-

| Acronym | Expanded Version |
|---|---|
| A1C | Glycated Hemoglobin A1C (also written HbA1c) — a blood test measuring average blood glucose over 2–3 months |
| HbA1c | Hemoglobin A1c — same as A1C; used interchangeably in the book |
| CGM | Continuous Glucose Monitor — a wearable sensor that measures glucose in interstitial fluid every few minutes |
| BMI | Body Mass Index — a measure of body fat based on height and |

| Acronym | Expanded Version |
| --- | --- |
| | weight (weight in kg / height in $m^2$) |
| GLP-1 | Glucagon-Like Peptide-1 — an incretin hormone; GLP-1 receptor agonists (are a class of diabetes/weight-loss medications |
| HIIT | High-Intensity Interval Training — alternating short bursts of intense exercise with recovery periods |
| DNA | Deoxyribonucleic Acid — genetic material; referenced in the context of how genetics influence glucose metabolism |
| T2D / Type 2 diabetes | Type 2 Diabetes — a metabolic condition characterized by insulin resistance and chronically elevated blood glucose |

| Acronym | Expanded Version |
|---|---|
| mg/dL | Milligrams per Deciliter — unit used to measure blood glucose concentration (standard in the US) |
| mmol/L | Millimoles per Liter — unit used to measure blood glucose concentration (standard outside the US) |
| TIR | Time in Range — the percentage of time CGM readings fall within a defined target glucose range |
| ADA | American Diabetes Association — cited for the prediabetes risk test |
| AHA | American Heart Association — cited for cardiovascular health resources |
| ACSM | American College of Sports Medicine — cited for exercise prescription guidelines |

| Acronym | Expanded Version |
|---|---|
| CDC | Centers for Disease Control and Prevention (US) — cited for BMI calculators and diabetes prevention resources |
| NAMI | National Alliance on Mental Illness — cited as a mental health resource |
| NHS | National Health Service (UK) — cited for the waist-to-height ratio calculator |
| NHLBI | National Heart, Lung, and Blood Institute (US) — cited for the NIH BMI calculator |
| NIH | National Institutes of Health (US) — cited for weight management resources |
| USDA | United States Department of Agriculture — cited for MyPlate nutrition guidance |

| Acronym | Expanded Version |
|---|---|
| WISEWOMAN | Well-Integrated Screening and Evaluation for Women Across the Nation — a CDC cardiovascular screening programme |
| YMCA | Young Men's Christian Association — referenced in the context of body fat calculator tools |
| JAMA | Journal of the American Medical Association — cited for the Leproult & Van Cauter (2010) sleep study |
| PubMed | PubMed — the NIH/NLM online database of biomedical literature; all citations in the book include PubMed links |
| STEP 4 | Semaglutide Treatment Effect in People with Obesity, Trial 4 — a clinical trial (Wilding et al., 2022, Diabetes Care) on GLP-1 receptor agonist maintenance therapy |

- 

**Medical Support**

Always consult with healthcare providers, especially if you have: - Existing diabetes or prediabetes - Other metabolic conditions - Are taking medications - Have questions about your specific health situation

**Disclaimer**: This book is for educational and informational purposes only and does not constitute medical advice. The author, Sudipta Mitra, is not a licensed medical doctor, registered dietitian, or certified diabetes educator. The information provided is based on research, published scientific literature, and the experiences of individuals using CGM technology for metabolic health and weight loss.

**Medical Consultation Required**: Always consult with qualified healthcare professionals before making significant changes to your diet, exercise routine, starting any monitoring program, or taking any supplements. Individual results may vary based on numerous factors including genetics, medical history, current health status, medications, and adherence to protocols.

**CGM Technology**: This book discusses the use of Continuous Glucose Monitors, which are medical devices. While CGMs are increasingly available for wellness purposes, they should be used under appropriate guidance. Follow all manufacturer instructions and consult healthcare providers if you have any concerns about your glucose levels or health.

**Not for Diabetes Management**: This book is intended for individuals without diabetes who are using CGM technology for metabolic optimization and weight loss. If you have diabetes, prediabetes, or any metabolic disorder, you must work exclusively with your healthcare team and follow their medical guidance. The protocols in this book may not be appropriate for individuals with these conditions.

**No Warranties**: The author and publisher make no representations or warranties of any kind regarding the completeness, accuracy, or suitability of the information contained in this book. All information is provided "as is" without warranty of any kind.

**Limitation of Liability**: In no event shall the author or publisher be liable for any direct, indirect, incidental, special, or consequential damages arising out of or in connection with the use of this book or the information contained herein.

**Individual Responsibility**: Readers assume full responsibility for their own health and well-being and for any decisions made based on information in this book. The author and publisher are not responsible for any adverse effects or consequences resulting from the use of any suggestions, protocols, or information described in this book.

**Product References**: References to specific CGM brands, apps, supplements, or other products are for informational purposes only and do not constitute endorsements. The author has no financial relationship with any companies mentioned unless specifically disclosed.

**Current Information**: Medical knowledge, technology, and best practices evolve constantly. Information in this book reflects knowledge available at the time of publication (2026) and may become outdated. Readers should verify information with current sources and healthcare providers.

## About the Author

Sudipta Mitra is not a doctor, nutritionist, or certified health coach—he's someone who got tired of failing at weight loss and decided to try something different.

After noticing significant metabolic changes in his 50s, Sudipta began experimenting with Continuous Glucose Monitor (CGM) technology to understand his body's unique responses to food. What started as a personal experiment became a transformative journey, resulting in 20 pounds lost in 3 months without calorie counting, deprivation, or confusion.

Through meticulous tracking and analysis of his own CGM data, Sudipta discovered that sustainable weight loss requires mastery of four interconnected dimensions: real-time metrics, strategic movement, sleep optimization, and stress management. His breakthrough insight was that these dimensions don't just add together—they multiply each other's effectiveness.

"The Glucose Reset" documents this journey and provides a framework for others to achieve their own transformations using data-driven, personalized approaches to health..

**For more information, updates, and resources, community visit:**

*https://www.facebook.com/igetreset/*

**Connect with the author:**

.

# Key Scientific References

# About This Book and Its Evidence

## Working Alongside Your Healthcare Team

The strategies in this book — food sequencing, post-meal movement, sleep, and glucose monitoring — are intended to complement professional medical care, not replace it. Please share what you discover with your doctor or dietitian. The data your CGM provides is genuinely useful clinical information, and your care team is best placed to help you act on it in the context of your full health picture.

## On GLP-1 Medications and This Book

GLP-1 receptor agonist medications —represent a genuine and exciting advance in metabolic medicine. For many people they have been life-changing, and this book has nothing but respect for the clinical work behind them and the physicians who prescribe them thoughtfully.

The lifestyle strategies in this book are designed to work alongside GLP-1 therapy, not instead of it. Food sequencing, post-meal movement, and glucose awareness engage many of the same metabolic pathways these medications support — and combining them can make both more effective. Research from the STEP 4 study (Wilding et al., 2022, Diabetes Care) highlights how important sustained lifestyle habits are for maintaining results over the long term, which is precisely what this book helps build. If your doctor has recommended GLP-1 medication, continuing that treatment while adopting the habits here is an excellent approach. Always make medication decisions in partnership with your physician.

## How Claims Are Made in This Book

The following describes how evidence is used and presented throughout this book.

- **Peer-reviewed citations.** Every major claim is supported by studies published in peer-reviewed journals including The Lancet, the New England Journal of Medicine, Diabetes Care, and Diabetologia. Full citations with direct PubMed links appear in the Key Scientific References section.
- **Hedged, accurate language.** Language is calibrated to the strength of the evidence. Strong, replicated findings are stated directly. Emerging or individual-variable findings are qualified with phrases such as "research suggests" or "in many individuals."
- **No brand names.** Guidance addresses food categories and behaviors rather than specific brands, keeping recommendations universally applicable.
- **Clear fact vs. opinion distinction.** Personal experience and interpretation are identified as such. Scientific findings are

presented with their source and scope stated.

- **Medical disclaimer.** A full medical disclaimer appears at the front of this book. Individual health decisions should always involve qualified professionals.

The citations in the Key Scientific References section are an open invitation to read the primary research yourself. Every study referenced is publicly available on PubMed.

The following peer-reviewed studies support key claims made in this book. Readers are encouraged to review primary sources and consult healthcare providers for guidance on their individual health circumstances.

## Sleep and Insulin Resistance

Spiegel, K., Leproult, R., & Van Cauter, E. (1999). Impact of sleep debt on metabolic and endocrine function. The Lancet, 354(9188), 1435–1439. [Sleep restriction of 6 nights to 4 hours reduced insulin sensitivity by ~30%.]

Donga, E., van Dijk, M., van Dijk, J. G., et al. (2010). A single night of partial sleep deprivation induces insulin resistance in multiple metabolic pathways in healthy subjects. Journal of Clinical Endocrinology & Metabolism, 95(6), 2963–2968.

## Post-Meal Exercise and Glucose Spikes

Colberg, S. R., Zarrabi, L., Bennington, L., et al. (2009). Postprandial walking is better for lowering the glycemic effect of dinner than pre-dinner exercise in type 2 diabetic individuals. Journal of the American Medical Directors Association, 10(6), 394–397.

Reynolds, A. N., Mann, J. I., Williams, S., & Venn, B. J. (2016). Advice to walk after meals is more effective for lowering postprandial glycaemia in type 2 diabetes mellitus than advice that does not specify timing: a randomized crossover study. Diabetologia, 59(12), 2572–2578.

## Food Sequencing and Glucose Response

Imai, S., Fukui, M., & Kajiyama, S. (2014). Effect of eating vegetables before carbohydrates on glucose excursions in patients with type 2 diabetes. Journal of Clinical Biochemistry and Nutrition, 54(1), 7–11. [Vegetable-first eating reduced glucose excursions by approximately 40%.]

Shukla, A. P., Iliescu, R. G., Thomas, C. E., & Aronne, L. J. (2017). Food order has a significant impact on postprandial glucose and insulin levels. Diabetes Care, 38(7), e98–e99.

## Diabetes Prevention

Knowler, W. C., Barrett-Connor, E., Fowler, S. E., et al. (2002). Reduction in the incidence of type 2 diabetes with lifestyle intervention or metformin. New England Journal of Medicine, 346(6), 393–403. [Lifestyle intervention reduced diabetes incidence by 58%; the source of the "50%" reduction claim.]

*Published 2026 First Edition*

Printed by Libri Plureos GmbH in Hamburg,
Germany

9 798994 952603